THE ULTIMATE GALVESTON DIET FOR BEGINNERS

1500 Days Of Low Carb, Anti-Inflammatory Recipes And Intermittent Fasting Diet Plan To Burn Fat And Tame Your Hormonal Symptoms

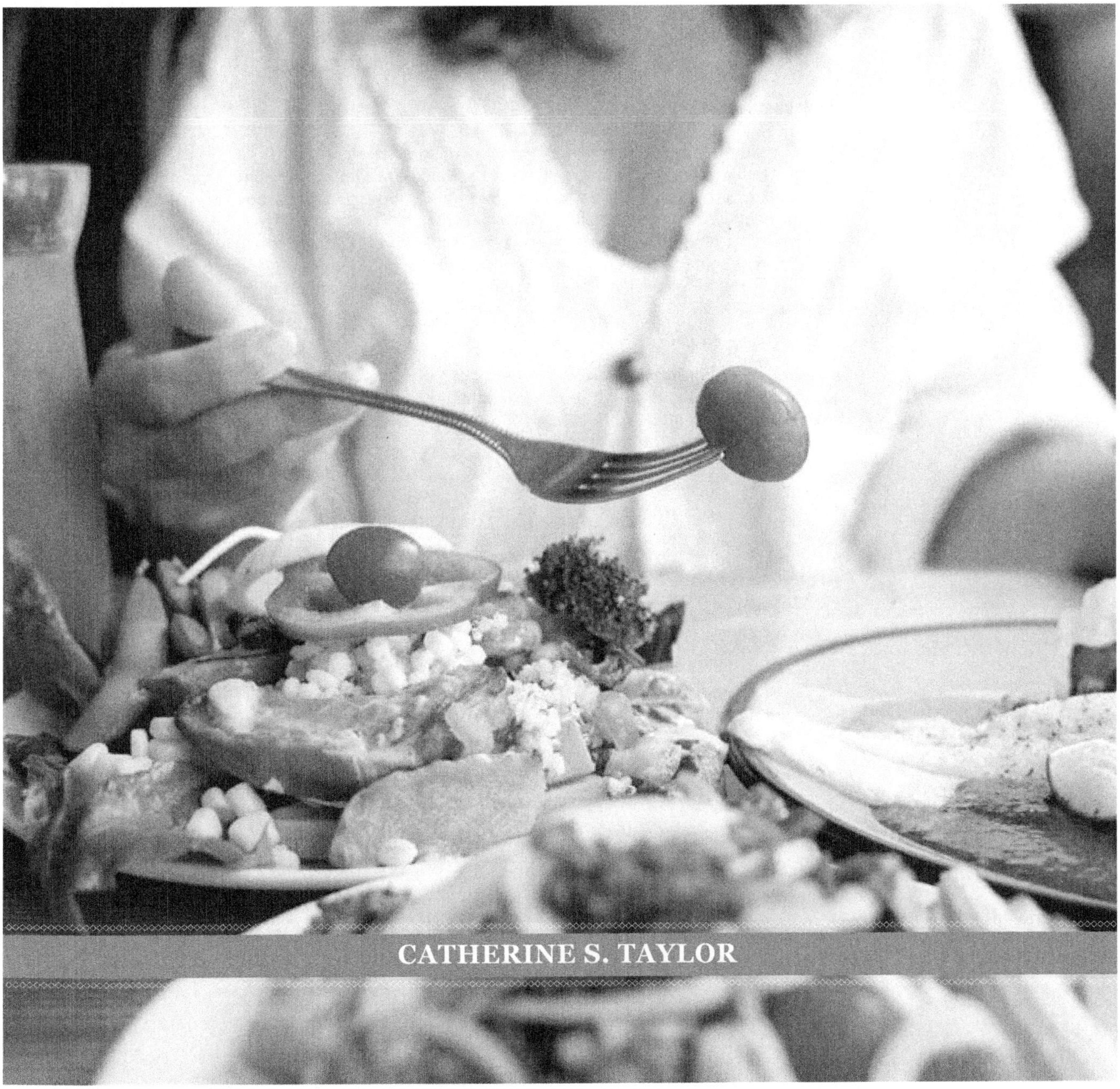

CATHERINE S. TAYLOR

Copyright© 2023 By Catherine S. Taylor Rights Reserved

This book is copyright protected. It is only for personal use. You cannot amend, distribute, sell, use, quote or paraphrase any part of the content within this book, without the consent of the author or publisher.

Under no circumstances will any blame or legal responsibility be held against the publisher, or author, for any damages, reparation, or monetary loss due to the information contained within this book, either directly or indirectly.

Disclaimer Notice:

Please note the information contained within this document is for educational and entertainment purposes only. All effort has been executed to present accurate, up to date, reliable, complete information. No warranties of any kind are declared or implied. Readers acknowledge that the author is not engaged in the rendering of legal, financial, medical or professional advice. The content within this book has been derived from various sources. Please consult a licensed professional before attempting any techniques outlined in this book.

By reading this document, the reader agrees that under no circumstances is the author responsible for any losses, direct or indirect, that are incurred as a result of the use of the information contained within this document, including, but not limited to, errors, omissions, or inaccuracies.

EDITOR: LYN	INTERIOR DESIGN: FAIZAN
COVER ART: ABR	FOOD STYLIST: JO

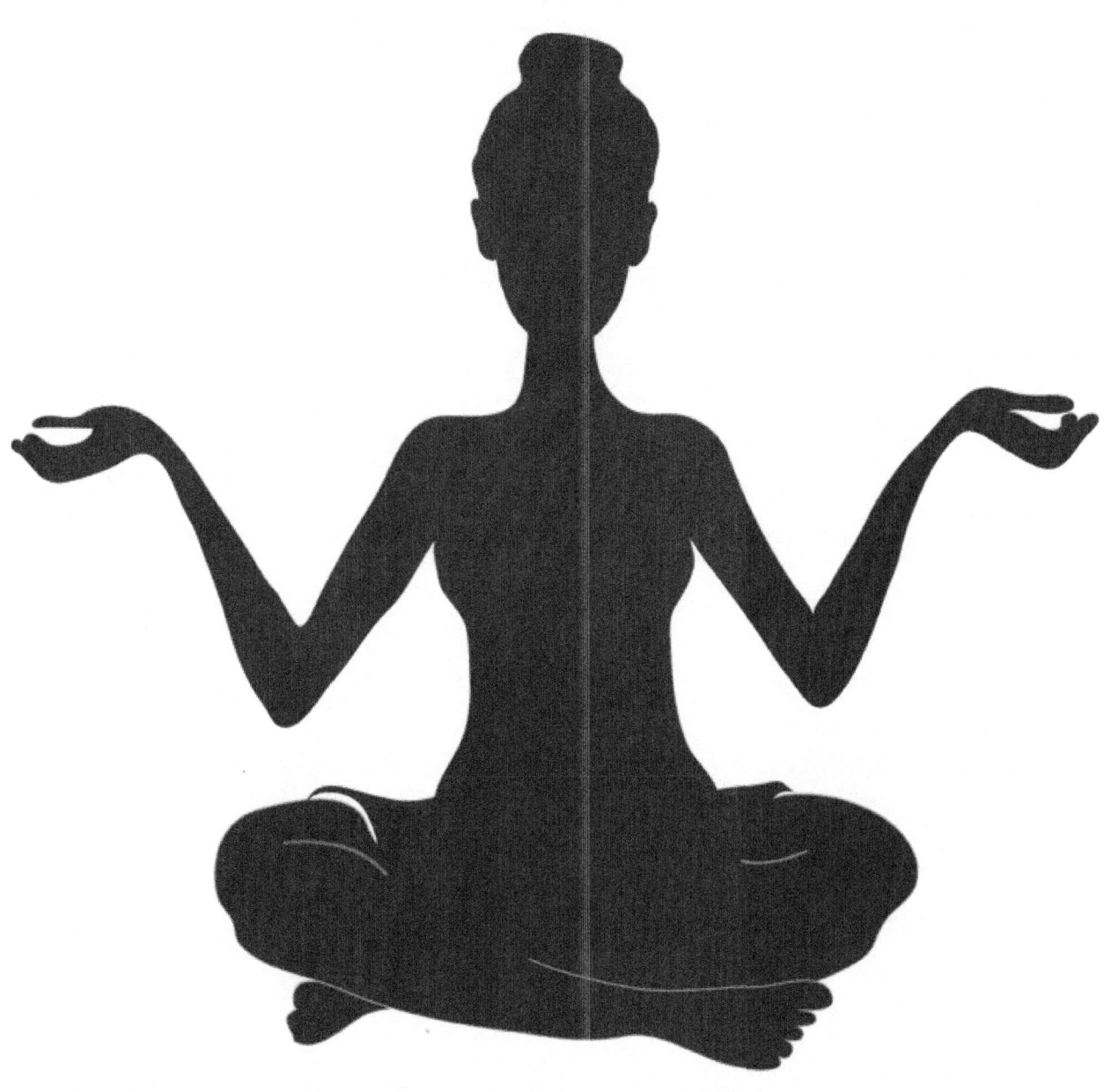

Table of Contents

Introduction ... 1

Chapter 1
Changes in midlife women ... 2
Perimenopause ... 3
Menopause ... 3
Postmenopause ... 3
Reasons for Midlife Women to Choose the Galveston Diet ... 4

Chapter 2
Galveston Diet Basics ... 5
The Principles of the Galveston Diet ... 6
The Science Behind the Galveston Diet ... 6
Explanation of Benefits of the Galveston Diet ... 8
Tips for Following the Galveston Diet ... 9
Foods to Include and Avoid on the Galveston Diet ... 9

Chapter 3
Start Your Galveston Diet Journal ... 10
Intermittent Fasting ... 11
Anti-Inflammatory Nutrition ... 11
Fuel Refocus ... 11
Q&A ... 12

Chapter 4
A Comprehensive Guide to Meal Planning ... 14
Tips for Planning and Preparing Meals on the Galveston Diet ... 15
Suggestions for Meal Prep and Batch Cooking ... 15

Chapter 5
The Meal Plans and Shopping Lists ... 16
The Conventional Menus: Week 1 ... 17
Shopping List for Week 1 ... 17
The Conventional Menus: Week 2 ... 17
Shopping List for Week 2 ... 18
The Conventional Menus: Week 3 ... 18
Shopping List for Week 3 ... 19
The Conventional Menus: Week 4 ... 19
Shopping List for Week 4 ... 19
The Vegetarian Menus: Week 1 ... 20
Shopping List for Vegetarian Week 1 ... 20
The Vegetarian Menus: Week 2 ... 20
Shopping List for Vegetarian Week 2 ... 21

Chapter 6
Smoothies & Breakfast ... 22
Tropical Papaya Smoothie ... 23
Chai Smoothie ... 23
Soothing Smoothie ... 23
Cleansing Smoothie ... 23
Watermelon Smoothie ... 24
Vegan Rib Roast ... 24
Morning Detox Smoothie ... 24
Olives Fritters ... 24
Mexican Muffins ... 25
Avocado Smoothie ... 25
Zucchini Hummus Wrap ... 25
Paprika Chips ... 25
Sea moss Banana Smoothie ... 26
Zucchini Crackers ... 26
Vegan Portobello Burgers ... 26
Mushroom Steak ... 27
Chard and Lime Pasta ... 27
Spiced Mushroom Bowl ... 28
Vegan Veggie Fritters ... 28

Chapter 7
Eggs ... 29
Reuben Egg Rolls ... 30
Spinach Eggs ... 30
Paprika Egg Cups ... 30
Basil Scotch Eggs ... 31
Eggs with Peppers ... 31
Chili Eggs ... 31
Spiced Eggs ... 31
Bacon-and-Eggs Avocado ... 32
Bacon and Spinach Egg Muffins ... 32
Cheddar Eggs ... 33
Baked Eggs ... 33
Classic Egg Sandwich ... 33
Spinach and Feta Egg Bake ... 34
Meritage Eggs ... 34
Scotch Eggs ... 34

Chapter 8
Soups & Stews ... 35
Gut-Healing Bone Broth ... 36
Garlic And Herb Vegetable Broth ... 36
Mexican Chicken Broth ... 36
Lemon Pepper Chicken Broth ... 37
Chayote Mushroom Stew ... 37
Zoodle Vegetable Soup ... 37
Thai Chicken Broth ... 37
Hungarian Beef Bone Broth ... 38
Miso Chicken Broth ... 38
Creamy Squash Soup ... 38
Chinese Pork Broth ... 38
Italian Tomato And Herb Beef Bone Broth ... 38
Pho Beef Bone Broth ... 38
Healthy Alkaline Green Soup ... 39
Butternut Pumpkin Soup ... 39
Spicy Soursop and Zucchini Soup ... 39
Zoodle Chickpea Soup ... 40
Kamut Squash Soup ... 40

Chapter 9
Salads & Sides ... 41
Zesty Citrus Salad ... 42
Kale and Sprouts Salad ... 42
Crunchy Zucchini Fries ... 42
Massaged Kale Salad ... 42
Peppery Rice Bowl ... 43
Spicy Sweet Potato Chips ... 43
Ginger Stir-Fried Pepper & Broccoli ... 43

Cinnamon & Ginger Apple Sautée	43
Basil and Avocado Salad	44
Swede & Carrot Purée	44
Delicious Chickpea & Mushroom Bowl	44
Catalan Spinach	44
Sage Sweet Potato Wedges	45
Chinese Trail Mix	45
Mexican Quinoa	45
Root-Veggie Chips	46
Grilled Romaine Lettuce Salad	46

Chapter 10
Vegan & Vegetarian — 47

Mixed Vegetable Stir-Fry	48
Cucumber and Basil Gazpacho	48
Vegetable Low Mein	48
Snap Peas Mash	48
Prosciutto Asparagus Mix	48
Thyme Radish Mix	49
Veggie Lettuce Wraps	49
Zucchini Linguine	49
Garlic Fennel Bulb	49
Paprika Asparagus	49
Power Pesto Zoodles	50
Roasted Squash and Apples	50
Mushroom Gravy	50
Chickpea and Kale Curry	50
Baked Portobello Mushrooms	51
Nori Burritos	51
Chickpea and Mushroom Curry	51
Spiced Okra Curry	51

Chapter 11
Seafood Dishes — 52

Tilapia Fish Tacos With Cilantro-Lime Crema	53
Whitefish With Spice Rub	53
Pecan-Crusted Trout	54
Sole with Vegetables in Foil Packets	54
Fish Sticks With Avocado Dipping Sauce	55
Sea Bass Baked with Tomatoes, Olives, and Capers	55
Smoked Trout Fried Rice	56
Open-Face Avocado Tuna Melts	56
Spiced Trout And Spinach	56
Mediterranean Baked Salmon	56
Grilled Salmon Packets With Asparagus	57
Dill Salmon With Cucumber-Radish Salad	57
Miso Baked Salmon	57
Quinoa Salmon Bowl	58
Salmon with Basil Gremolata	58
Salmon & Asparagus Skewers	58
Coconut-Crusted Cod With Mango-Pineapple Salsa	59
Curried Poached Halibut	59

Chapter 12
Poultry & Meat Dishes — 60

Turkey Larb Lettuce Wraps	61
Indonesian Chicken Satay	61
Brown Rice Congee	61
Turkey Chili	62
Apple-Turkey Burgers	62
Glazed Chicken With Broccoli	62
Turkey-Thyme Meatballs	62
Slow-Cooker Chicken Alfredo	63
Lamb-Stuffed Peppers	63
Baked Turkey Meatballs With Zucchini Noodles	63
Coconut Chicken Curry	63
Chicken Sliders	64
Sesame Chicken Stir-Fry	64
Lamb Souvlaki	64
Coconut-Braised Chicken	64
Chicken Buckwheat Florentine	65
Bubbie'S Comforting Chicken Soup	65
Pork Tenderloin With Savory Berry Sauce	65
Pork Chops With Cooked Apple Salsa	66
Grainy Mustard-Crusted Lamb	66
Moroccan Lamb Stew	67
Savory Beef Meatloaf	67
Buckwheat Cabbage Rolls	67

Chapter 13
Snacks, Appetizers, and Savory Fat Bombs — 68

Mushroom Bites	69
Roasted Garlic Mushrooms	69
Smoked Almonds	69
Banana "Nice" Cream	69
Mediterranean Cucumber Bites	70
Parmesan Zucchini Chips	70
Roasted Cauliflower Hummus	70
No-Fail Deviled Eggs	70
Flaxseed Chips And Guacamole	71
Zucchini Fritters	71
Cheesy Crackers	71
Caprese Stuffed Avocados	72
Baked Olives	72
Savory Party Mix	72
Three-Cheese Stuffed Mushrooms	72
Creamy Spinach Dip	73
Herbed Mozzarella Sticks	73
Cheesy Cauliflower Breadsticks	73

Appendix 1 Measurement Conversion Chart	74
Appendix 2 The Dirty Dozen and Clean Fifteen	75
Appendix 3 Index	76

Introduction

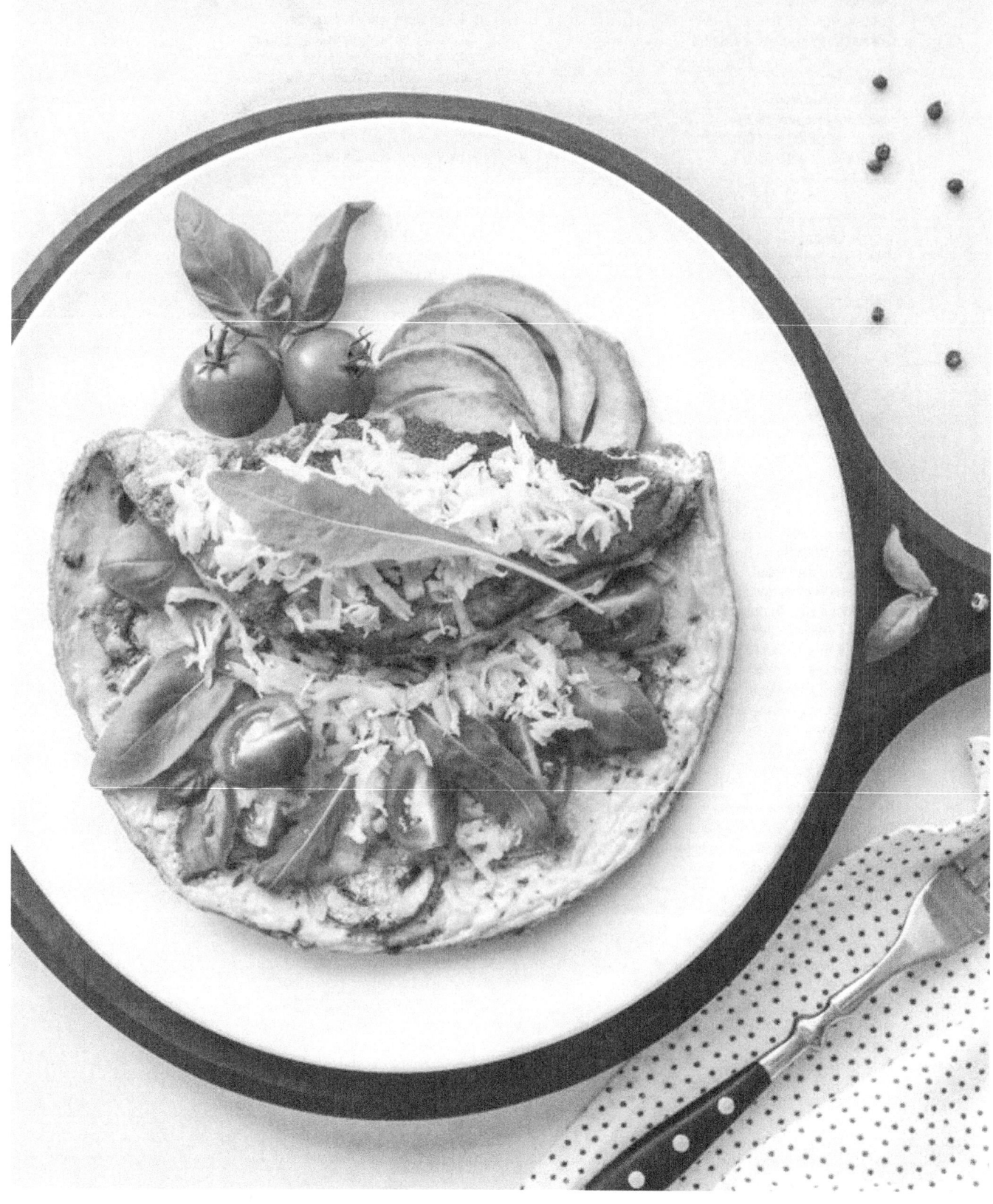

The Galveston diet is a revolutionary approach to weight loss and optimal health that has been gaining traction in recent years. This unique dietary plan was developed by Dr. Mary Claire Haver, a renowned OB-GYN and hormone expert, after years of researching the relationship between hormones, weight loss, and overall health.

At its core, the Galveston diet is a plant-based, low-carbohydrate eating plan that is designed to support healthy hormone function, balance blood sugar levels, and promote long-term weight loss. Unlike many other diets that focus on calorie counting or extreme restrictions, the Galveston diet is based on real, whole foods that are nourishing and satisfying.

The Galveston diet has been shown to be effective for a wide range of individuals, from women experiencing menopause-related weight gain to athletes seeking to improve their performance and recovery. By emphasizing nutrient-dense foods that support hormone function, the Galveston diet can help to address a range of health issues, including inflammation, insulin resistance, and hormonal imbalances.

This cookbook is designed to help you implement the principles of the Galveston diet in your own life, with delicious and satisfying recipes that are easy to prepare and full of flavor. Whether you're looking for healthy breakfast options, quick and easy snacks, or delicious main dishes that the whole family will love, this cookbook has something for everyone.

Each recipe in this cookbook is based on the principles of the Galveston diet, with a focus on nutrient-dense ingredients that support hormone function and overall health. From hearty salads and bowls to satisfying main dishes and indulgent desserts, you'll find plenty of inspiration for creating delicious and healthy meals that nourish your body and satisfy your taste buds.

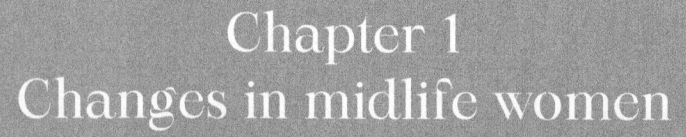

Chapter 1
Changes in midlife women

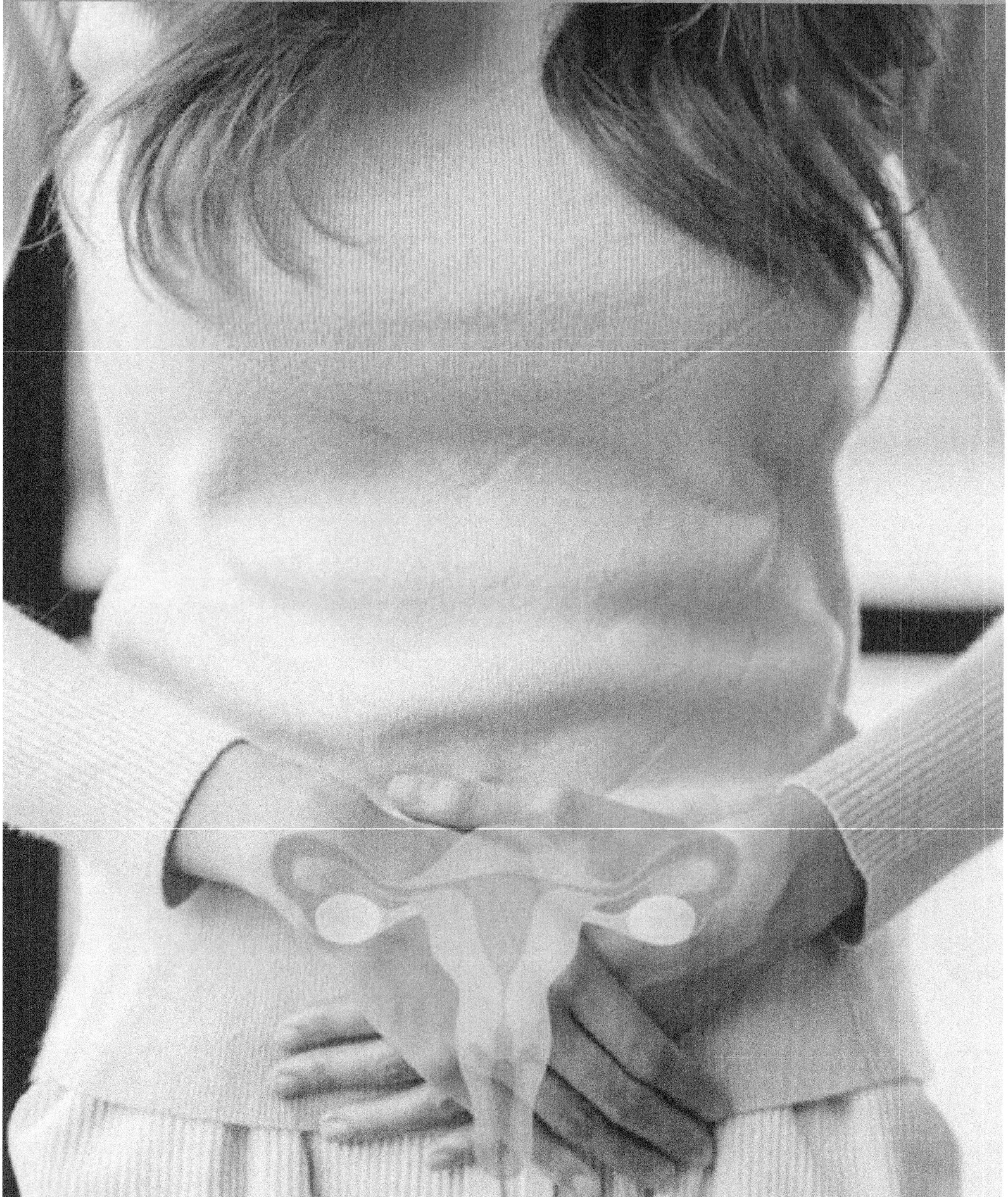

Perimenopause

Perimenopause is the first stage of hormonal fluctuation that occurs in women as they approach menopause. It is a transitional phase that begins several years before menopause, typically in a woman's 40s but can start earlier or later for some women. Perimenopause can last anywhere from a few months to several years, and during this time, the body undergoes various hormonal changes that can result in a range of symptoms.

During perimenopause, the ovaries begin to produce less estrogen, which is the hormone responsible for regulating the menstrual cycle and supporting fertility. As estrogen levels fluctuate, women may experience irregular periods, hot flashes, night sweats, and other symptoms that are commonly associated with menopause. Perimenopause can also affect mood, sleep, and energy levels, leading to feelings of fatigue, irritability, and depression.

Perimenopause is the period of transition that occurs before menopause. During this time, the levels of estrogen and other hormones fluctuate, which can lead to a range of symptoms. Here are some of the common symptoms of perimenopause and their explanations:

1. Irregular periods: One of the first signs of perimenopause is changes in menstrual cycles. The periods may become shorter or longer, lighter or heavier, and more or less frequent. This is due to the fluctuation in hormone levels.
2. Hot flashes and night sweats: Hot flashes are a sudden feeling of warmth that spreads over the body, especially the face and neck. They can be accompanied by sweating and palpitations. Night sweats are similar, but occur during sleep. These symptoms are caused by the hormonal changes in the body.
3. Mood changes: Perimenopause can cause mood swings, irritability, anxiety, and depression. These changes can be attributed to the hormonal imbalances in the body.
4. Vaginal dryness: As estrogen levels decrease, the tissues in the vagina may become dry and less elastic. This can cause discomfort, itching, and pain during sex.
5. Sleep disturbances: Many women experience sleep disturbances during perimenopause, including insomnia and waking up frequently during the night. These symptoms are caused by hot flashes, night sweats, and other hormonal changes.
6. Decreased fertility: As women approach menopause, their fertility declines. It may become harder to get pregnant and the risk of miscarriage increases.
7. Changes in sexual function: Perimenopause can cause a decrease in libido, as well as changes in sexual function such as difficulty achieving orgasm.
8. Fatigue: Many women experience fatigue and a lack of energy during perimenopause. This is likely due to the hormonal changes and sleep disturbances that occur.
9. Changes in skin and hair: Hormonal changes can cause changes in the skin and hair, including dryness, thinning, and loss of elasticity.

Menopause

Menopause is a natural biological process that marks the end of a woman's reproductive years. It is defined as the permanent cessation of menstrual periods for at least 12 consecutive months due to a decline in hormone production by the ovaries.

Perimenopause is the transitional phase that precedes menopause, during which the ovaries gradually produce less estrogen, leading to irregular periods, hot flashes, night sweats, vaginal dryness, and other symptoms. Perimenopause can last anywhere from a few months to several years, and it usually starts in a woman's 40s but can occur earlier or later.

Once a woman has gone without a menstrual period for 12 consecutive months, she has reached menopause. At this point, the ovaries have stopped releasing eggs, and hormone levels, including estrogen, are significantly lower than during a woman's reproductive years. As a result, women may experience a variety of symptoms, such as hot flashes, night sweats, vaginal dryness, mood changes, and decreased sex drive.

It's important to note that menopause is a natural and inevitable part of aging, and it's not a disease or a medical condition that needs to be treated. However, some women may choose to seek medical advice or treatment to alleviate their symptoms and maintain their overall health and well-being during this transition.

Postmenopause

Postmenopause is the stage of life that begins after a woman has gone without a menstrual period for 12 consecutive months or longer. At this point, the hormonal changes associated with menopause have typically stabilized, and most menopausal symptoms have subsided. However, women may still be at increased risk for certain health conditions, such as osteoporosis and cardiovascular disease, due to the decline in estrogen levels that occurs during and after menopause. It's important for women to continue to prioritize their health and well-being during postmenopause by eating a healthy diet, exercising regularly, getting regular health checkups, and seeking medical advice if they experience any concerning symptoms.

Reasons for Midlife Women to Choose the Galveston Diet

Midlife women refer to women who are in their middle age, typically between the ages of 40 and 60. This period of life can be characterized by many changes, both physically and emotionally, including menopause, changes in hormone levels, aging-related health concerns, and life transitions such as children leaving home or retirement.

During this time, it's important for midlife women to focus on their health and well-being to prevent or manage chronic health conditions that can develop later in life. This includes maintaining a healthy diet, exercising regularly, getting enough sleep, and managing stress.

One diet that has gained attention for its potential health benefits for midlife women is the Galveston diet. This is a low-carbohydrate, high-healthy fat diet that was developed by Dr. Mary Claire Haver, a board-certified OBGYN who specializes in menopause and hormonal health.

The Galveston diet emphasizes whole foods such as fruits, vegetables, nuts, seeds, and healthy fats, and limits processed and refined carbohydrates. It also includes intermittent fasting, which involves restricting food intake to certain windows of time each day.

The diet aims to balance hormones and reduce inflammation, which can help alleviate symptoms of menopause and reduce the risk of chronic health conditions such as heart disease, diabetes, and cancer. However, as with any diet, it's important to consult with a healthcare professional before starting the Galveston diet or any other dietary changes.

In summary, midlife women face many physical and emotional changes, and it's important for them to prioritize their health and well-being during this time. The Galveston diet is one potential dietary approach that may offer health benefits for midlife women, but it's important to consult with a healthcare professional before making any dietary changes.

The Galveston Diet is designed specifically for midlife women, particularly those in perimenopause and menopause, and it can be beneficial in several ways:

1. Hormone balance: Women in perimenopause and menopause experience significant changes in hormone levels, which can lead to weight gain, mood swings, and other symptoms. The Galveston Diet focuses on nutrient-dense, whole foods that can help to support hormone balance, reducing symptoms like hot flashes, night sweats, and mood swings.
2. Weight management: Many women in midlife struggle with weight gain and find it harder to lose weight. The Galveston Diet promotes a whole-foods approach to eating that is high in protein, healthy fats, and fiber, which can help to keep women feeling fuller for longer and support healthy weight management.
3. Reduced inflammation: Chronic inflammation has been linked to a number of health problems, including heart disease, diabetes, and cancer. The Galveston Diet emphasizes anti-inflammatory foods, such as fatty fish, berries, dark leafy greens, nuts, seeds, and turmeric, which can help to reduce inflammation in the body.
4. Improved energy and mood: Many women in midlife experience fatigue and mood swings, which can be exacerbated by poor nutrition. The Galveston Diet promotes a whole-foods approach to eating that can help to improve energy levels and stabilize mood.
5. Reduced risk of chronic disease: Women in midlife are at an increased risk for chronic diseases, such as heart disease, diabetes, and cancer. The Galveston Diet emphasizes a nutrient-dense, whole-foods approach to eating that can help to reduce the risk of these diseases by promoting healthy weight management, reducing inflammation, and supporting overall health.

Chapter 2
Galveston Diet Basics

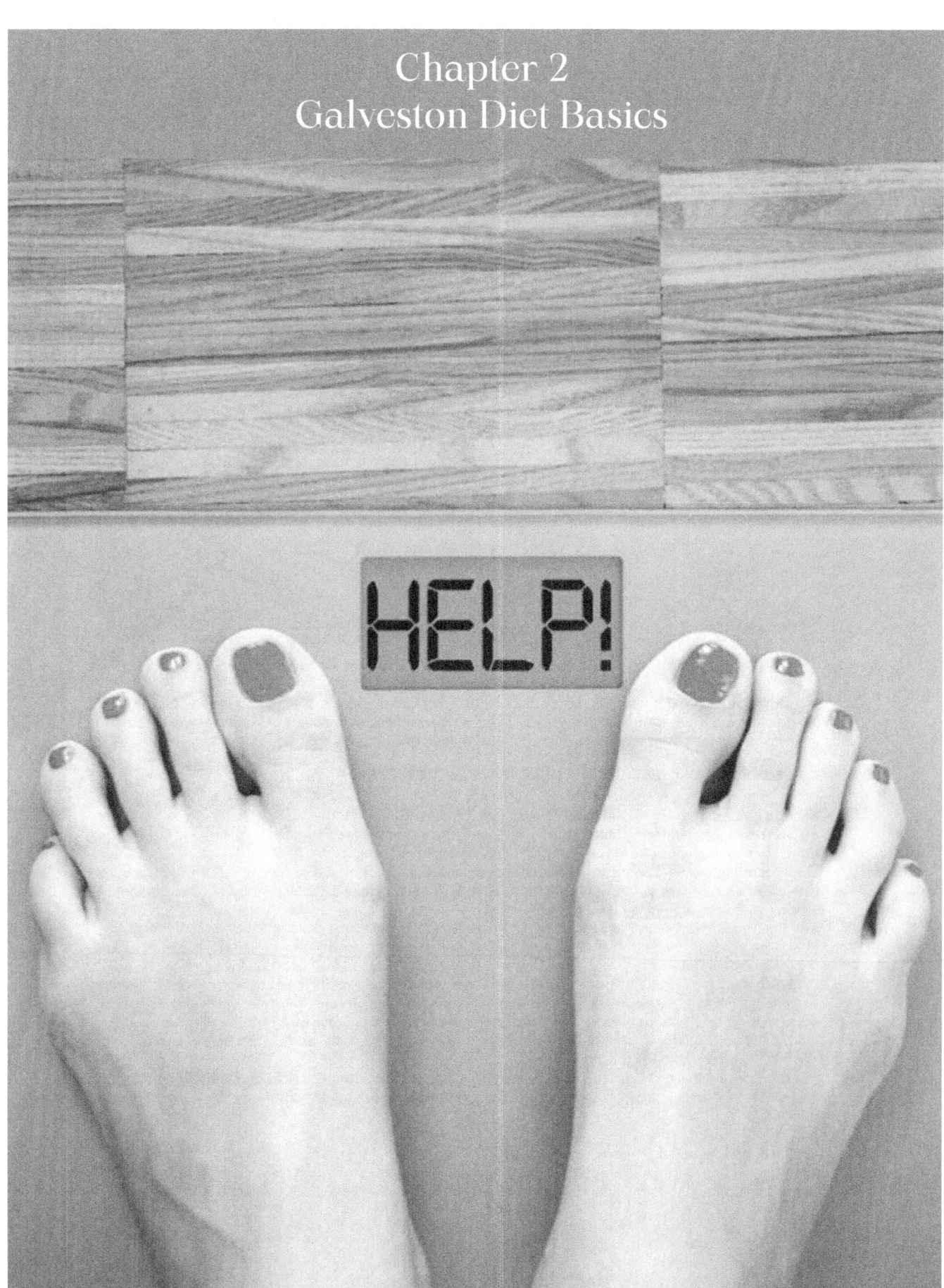

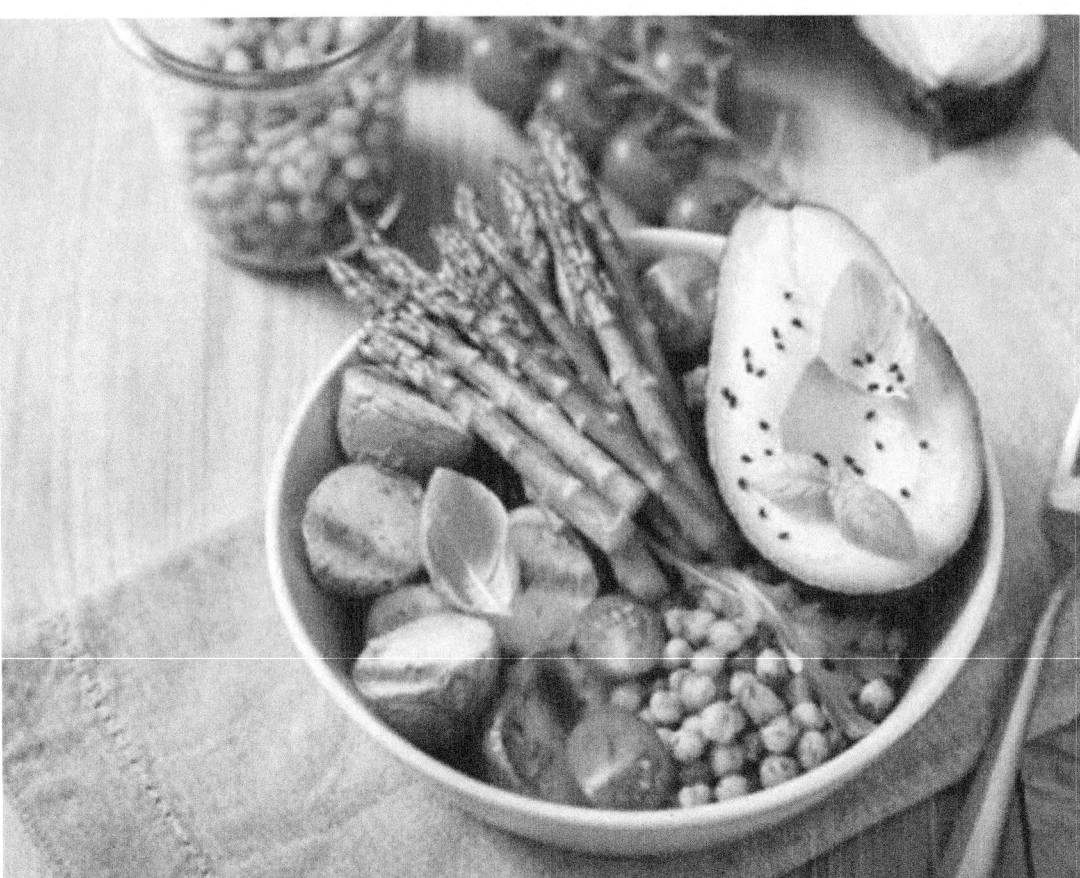

The Principles of the Galveston Diet

The Galveston diet is a weight loss program created by Dr. Mary Claire Haver, a board-certified obstetrician and gynecologist. The principles of the Galveston diet are based on research in the fields of endocrinology, nutrition, and metabolism, and are designed to help individuals lose weight and improve their overall health.

SOME OF THE KEY PRINCIPLES OF THE GALVESTON DIET INCLUDE:

1. Balancing hormones: The Galveston diet is designed to help balance hormones, particularly in women over 40 who may be experiencing hormonal changes. The diet includes foods that can help regulate insulin and other hormones, such as lean protein, healthy fats, and fiber-rich vegetables.
2. Eating nutrient-dense foods: The Galveston diet emphasizes nutrient-dense foods that provide the body with the vitamins, minerals, and antioxidants it needs to function optimally. These include fruits, vegetables, whole grains, lean protein, and healthy fats.
3. Avoiding processed foods: The Galveston diet encourages individuals to avoid processed foods, which are often high in sugar, unhealthy fats, and additives. Instead, the diet emphasizes whole, natural foods that are minimally processed.
4. Eating according to a schedule: The Galveston diet encourages individuals to eat according to a schedule, with regular meals and snacks throughout the day. This can help regulate blood sugar and prevent overeating.
5. Incorporating intermittent fasting: The Galveston diet includes periods of intermittent fasting, where individuals limit their food intake for a certain period of time each day or week. This can help improve insulin sensitivity and promote weight loss.
6. Drinking plenty of water: The Galveston diet emphasizes the importance of staying hydrated by drinking plenty of water throughout the day. This can help support digestion, regulate body temperature, and promote healthy skin.

The Science Behind the Galveston Diet

The science behind the Galveston diet is based on several principles that have been studied and shown to have potential benefits for weight loss and metabolic health. These principles include:

Low-carbohydrate, high-fat (LCHF) diet: The Galveston diet is a low-carbohydrate, high-fat diet that focuses on whole, unprocessed foods. LCHF diets have been shown to be effective for weight loss, improving blood sugar control, and reducing inflammation. The Galveston diet emphasizes healthy fats, such as olive oil, avocado, nuts, and seeds, while limiting carbohydrates, including sugar, refined grains, and starchy vegetables.

The Galveston diet emphasizes a moderate intake of protein, a high intake of healthy fats, and a low intake of carbohydrates. Women following the diet are encouraged to consume a variety of nutrient-dense, whole foods, including lean meats, fish, poultry, eggs, nuts, seeds, healthy oils, and plenty of non-starchy vegetables. The diet also allows for some fruit and dairy, but these should be consumed in moderation.

The Galveston diet is a low-carbohydrate diet, which means that women following the diet are encouraged to limit their intake of refined carbohydrates, such as white bread, pasta, and sugary snacks. Instead, the diet emphasizes carbohydrates from whole, unprocessed sources, such as vegetables, fruits, and whole grains. By reducing carbohydrate intake and increasing fat intake, the body is encouraged to use fat as a primary source of energy, a process known as ketosis.

The Galveston diet also encourages women to focus on whole, unprocessed foods, rather than relying on packaged or convenience foods that are often high in calories, sugar, and unhealthy fats. By consuming whole, nutrient-dense foods, women can ensure that they are getting the vitamins, minerals, and other nutrients their bodies need to function properly.

Overall, the Galveston diet is a low-carbohydrate, high-fat diet that focuses on whole, unprocessed foods. By emphasizing healthy fats, moderate protein, and limited carbohydrates, the diet can help women manage their weight, improve their overall health, and reduce symptoms associated with perimenopause and menopause.

Ketogenic diet: The Galveston diet is similar to the ketogenic diet, which is a very low-carbohydrate, high-fat diet that has been shown to promote weight loss and improve metabolic health. The Galveston diet includes foods that are also common on a ketogenic diet, such as high-fat dairy, meat, fish, and eggs.

The Galveston diet shares some similarities with the ketogenic diet, which is a very low-carbohydrate, high-fat diet that has gained popularity in recent years. Like the Galveston diet, the ketogenic diet emphasizes a low intake of carbohydrates and a high intake of healthy fats.

However, there are some differences between the two diets. The ketogenic diet typically involves restricting carbohydrate intake to less than 20-50 grams per day, which can be challenging for some people to maintain. The Galveston diet allows for a higher intake of carbohydrates, with an emphasis on whole, unprocessed sources of carbohydrates such as vegetables, fruits, and whole grains.

The Galveston diet also places a greater emphasis on protein intake than the ketogenic diet. Women following the Galveston diet are encouraged to consume a moderate amount of protein, which can help to support muscle maintenance and repair.

Additionally, the Galveston diet is specifically designed for women in perimenopause and menopause, whereas the ketogenic diet is not targeted to a specific demographic. The Galveston diet takes into account the unique nutritional needs of women in midlife, who may be experiencing hormonal changes and associated symptoms such as weight gain and mood swings.

Overall, while the Galveston diet shares some similarities with the ketogenic diet, it is a more moderate approach that is specifically tailored to the nutritional needs of midlife women. By emphasizing a low intake of refined carbohydrates, a high intake of healthy fats, and a moderate intake of protein from whole, unprocessed sources, the Galveston diet can help women in perimenopause and menopause manage their weight, improve their overall health, and reduce symptoms associated with hormonal changes.

Whole, unprocessed foods: The Galveston diet emphasizes whole, unprocessed foods, which are generally more nutrient-dense than processed foods. The Galveston diet encourages the consumption of whole foods such as vegetables, fruits, nuts, and seeds.

The Galveston diet places a strong emphasis on consuming whole, unprocessed foods, rather than relying on packaged or processed foods. Whole, unprocessed foods are generally more nutrient-dense than processed foods, meaning they contain a higher concentration of vitamins, minerals, and other essential nutrients that the body needs to function properly.

When foods are processed, they often lose some of their nutritional value. For example, processed grains, such as white flour, have been stripped of their bran and germ, which contain most of the fiber, vitamins, and minerals. This leaves behind a starchy, refined carbohydrate that is quickly absorbed by the body and can lead to blood sugar spikes and crashes.

In contrast, whole grains, such as brown rice or quinoa, contain all parts of the grain, including the bran and germ, which provide a wealth of nutrients and fiber. This makes them a more nutrient-dense choice that can help to stabilize blood sugar and promote feelings of fullness and satisfaction.

Similarly, fruits and vegetables that are fresh and unprocessed are generally higher in vitamins, minerals, and phytonutrients than those that are canned or processed. Canned fruits and vegetables are often packed in syrup or loaded with added salt, which can be detrimental to health.

By emphasizing whole, unprocessed foods, the Galveston diet encourages women to choose foods that are more nutrient-dense and less processed. This can help to ensure that they are getting the vitamins, minerals, and other nutrients their bodies need to function properly, while also supporting overall health and wellbeing.

Protein intake: The Galveston diet encourages protein intake from animal sources, such as meat, fish, and eggs, which can help promote satiety and preserve muscle mass during weight loss. The Galveston diet includes protein-rich foods such as chicken, fish, beef, and pork.

The Galveston diet encourages a moderate intake of protein from whole, unprocessed sources, including animal sources such as meat, fish, and eggs. Protein is an essential macronutrient that is important for maintaining and repairing muscle tissue, as well as promoting feelings of fullness and satiety.

When people are trying to lose weight, it's important to preserve muscle mass, as this can help to support a healthy metabolism and prevent weight regain. Protein plays an important role in this, as it helps to preserve muscle mass while the body is in a calorie deficit.

Animal sources of protein are particularly beneficial in this regard, as they contain all of the essential amino acids needed to support muscle maintenance and repair. In addition, animal protein is generally more satiating than plant-based protein, which can help to promote feelings of fullness and reduce the likelihood of overeating.

However, it's important to note that the Galveston diet does not encourage excessive protein intake, as this can put a strain on the kidneys and other organs. Rather, the diet emphasizes a moderate intake of protein, along with plenty of healthy fats and whole, unprocessed sources of carbohydrates.

Overall, by encouraging a moderate intake of protein from animal sources, the Galveston diet can help women to preserve muscle mass and promote feelings of fullness and satiety during weight loss, while also providing a variety of essential nutrients and supporting overall health and wellbeing.

Explanation of Benefits of the Galveston Diet

The Galveston diet is a weight loss program that has several potential benefits, based on the principles of low-carbohydrate, high-fat diets and whole, unprocessed foods. These benefits include:

Weight loss: The Galveston diet can promote weight loss by reducing carbohydrate intake and increasing fat and protein intake, which can help increase feelings of fullness and reduce overall calorie intake.

Improved blood sugar control: The Galveston diet may help improve blood sugar control by reducing carbohydrate intake, which can lower blood sugar and insulin levels. This may be especially beneficial for individuals with insulin resistance or type 2 diabetes.

Reduced inflammation: The Galveston diet emphasizes whole, unprocessed foods that are rich in anti-inflammatory nutrients, such as fiber, vitamins, and minerals. This can help reduce inflammation throughout the body, which is associated with a range of chronic diseases.

Improved cholesterol levels: The Galveston diet may help improve cholesterol levels by increasing intake of healthy fats, such as monounsaturated and polyunsaturated fats, which can help raise HDL (the "good" cholesterol) and lower LDL (the "bad" cholesterol).

Reduced risk of heart disease: The Galveston diet may help reduce the risk of heart disease by improving cholesterol levels, reducing inflammation, and promoting weight loss.

Improved energy levels: The Galveston diet can provide sustained energy throughout the day by reducing fluctuations in blood sugar levels and promoting the use of fat for fuel instead of carbohydrates.
However, it is important to note that the Galveston diet may not be suitable for everyone, and it is important to speak with a healthcare provider before starting any new diet or weight loss program. Additionally, the long-term effects of the Galveston diet are not well understood and more research is needed to fully understand its potential benefits and risks.

Tips for Following the Galveston Diet

IF YOU ARE CONSIDERING FOLLOWING THE GALVESTON DIET, HERE ARE SOME TIPS TO HELP YOU GET STARTED:

1. Educate yourself: Before starting the Galveston diet, educate yourself about the principles behind the diet and the types of foods you should be eating. This can help you make informed choices and ensure you are following the diet correctly.
2. Plan your meals: Planning your meals in advance can help ensure you have the right foods on hand and can avoid making impulsive choices. Consider meal prepping or using a meal delivery service to make meal planning easier.
3. Focus on whole, unprocessed foods: The Galveston diet emphasizes whole, unprocessed foods, such as vegetables, fruits, nuts, seeds, and healthy fats. Aim to make these foods the foundation of your diet.
4. Limit carbohydrates: The Galveston diet is low in carbohydrates, so aim to limit your intake of sugar, refined grains, and starchy vegetables. Instead, focus on non-starchy vegetables and low-carbohydrate fruits.
5. Increase healthy fat intake: The Galveston diet encourages the consumption of healthy fats, such as olive oil, avocado, nuts, and seeds. Aim to include these foods in your meals and snacks.
6. Monitor protein intake: While the Galveston diet encourages protein intake, it is important to monitor your intake and make sure you are not consuming too much protein, which can be harmful to your kidneys.
7. Stay hydrated: Drinking plenty of water can help you stay hydrated and feel full throughout the day. Aim to drink at least 8 cups of water per day.
8. Get enough fiber: Fiber is important for digestive health and can help you feel full. Aim to include high-fiber foods, such as vegetables, fruits, and nuts, in your diet.
9. Exercise regularly: Regular exercise can help you lose weight, build muscle, and improve your overall health. Aim to get at least 30 minutes of moderate-intensity exercise most days of the week.
10. Consult with a healthcare provider: Before starting the Galveston diet or any new diet or weight loss program, it is important to consult with a healthcare provider to ensure it is safe and appropriate for your individual needs.

Foods to Include and Avoid on the Galveston Diet

The Galveston diet emphasizes whole, unprocessed foods, low carbohydrates and high fat intake. Here are some foods to include and avoid when following the Galveston diet:

FOODS TO INCLUDE:

- Non-starchy vegetables such as spinach, broccoli, cauliflower, bell peppers, asparagus, and zucchini.
- Low-carbohydrate fruits such as berries, avocados, and tomatoes.
- Healthy fats such as olive oil, coconut oil, avocado, nuts, and seeds.
- Proteins such as chicken, turkey, beef, lamb, fish, eggs, and tofu.
- Dairy products such as cheese, yogurt, and butter (in moderation).

FOODS TO AVOID:

- High-carbohydrate foods such as bread, pasta, rice, potatoes, and sugary snacks.
- Processed foods such as chips, crackers, and packaged meals.
- Sweetened beverages such as soda, fruit juice, and sports drinks.
- Artificial sweeteners and sugar alcohols.
- Excessive alcohol intake.

Chapter 3
Start Your Galveston Diet Journal

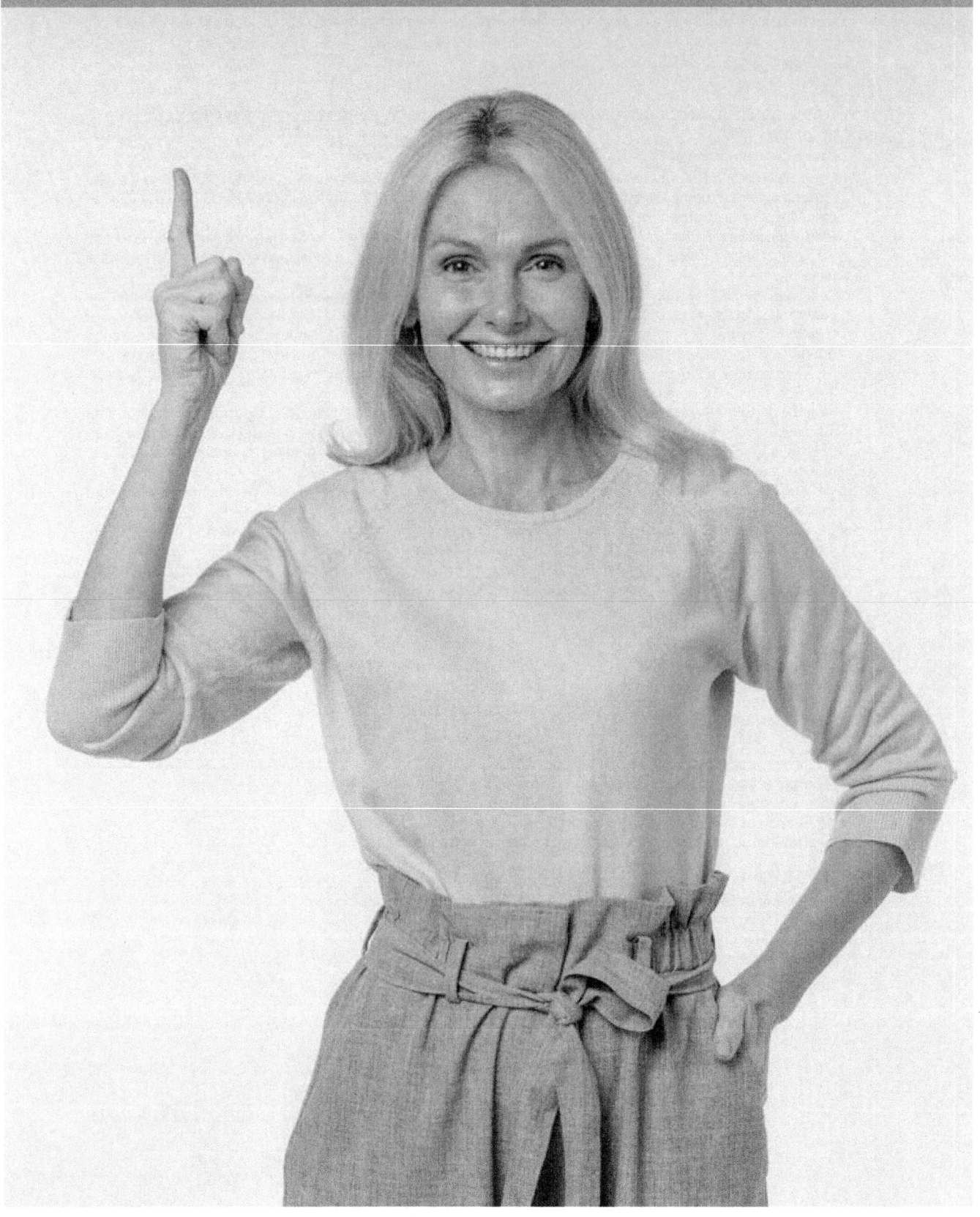

Intermittent Fasting

The Galveston Diet is a nutrition and weight loss program designed specifically for women who are in perimenopause or menopause. It was created by Dr. Mary Claire Haver, an obstetrician-gynecologist who experienced her own struggles with weight gain and hormone-related health issues. One aspect of the Galveston Diet is intermittent fasting.

Intermittent fasting involves restricting food intake for certain periods of time, alternating with periods of normal or increased food intake. The Galveston Diet recommends a 16:8 fasting protocol, which means fasting for 16 hours and having an 8-hour eating window each day.

During the fasting period, no calories are consumed, although water, black coffee, and other non-caloric beverages are allowed. The eating window can be adjusted to suit individual needs and preferences, but it is typically recommended to consume two to three meals within the 8-hour window.

Intermittent fasting has been shown to have a number of health benefits, including weight loss, improved insulin sensitivity, and reduced inflammation. It may also help with hormone balance, which is particularly important for women going through perimenopause and menopause.

However, it is important to note that intermittent fasting may not be suitable for everyone, particularly those with certain medical conditions or who are pregnant or breastfeeding. It is important to talk to a healthcare provider before starting any new diet or exercise program, including intermittent fasting.

Anti-Inflammatory Nutrition

Anti-inflammatory nutrition is a key component of the Galveston Diet, which is designed to help women in perimenopause and menopause manage their weight and improve their overall health. Inflammation is a natural response of the body to injury or infection, but chronic inflammation has been linked to a number of health problems, including heart disease, diabetes, and cancer. Anti-inflammatory nutrition aims to reduce chronic inflammation in the body by promoting the consumption of foods that are high in anti-inflammatory compounds and avoiding foods that promote inflammation.

The Galveston Diet recommends a diet that is rich in whole, minimally processed foods, such as fruits, vegetables, whole grains, lean proteins, and healthy fats. These foods are naturally anti-inflammatory, as they contain vitamins, minerals, and phytonutrients that can help to reduce inflammation in the body.

SOME SPECIFIC ANTI-INFLAMMATORY FOODS THAT ARE RECOMMENDED ON THE GALVESTON DIET INCLUDE:

1. Fatty fish, such as salmon and tuna, which are high in omega-3 fatty acids.
2. Berries, such as blueberries and raspberries, which are rich in antioxidants and other anti-inflammatory compounds.
3. Dark leafy greens, such as kale and spinach, which are high in vitamins and minerals that can help to reduce inflammation.
4. Nuts and seeds, such as almonds and flaxseeds, which are high in healthy fats and other anti-inflammatory nutrients.
5. Turmeric, which is a spice that contains curcumin, a potent anti-inflammatory compound.

On the other hand, the Galveston Diet recommends avoiding foods that are known to promote inflammation, such as processed foods, refined carbohydrates, sugary drinks, and foods high in saturated and trans fats.
By following an anti-inflammatory diet, women on the Galveston Diet may be able to reduce chronic inflammation in the body, which can improve their overall health and reduce their risk of chronic diseases.

Fuel Refocus

Fuel Refocus is another important aspect of the Galveston Diet, which is designed to help women in perimenopause and menopause manage their weight and improve their overall health. Fuel Refocus is a concept that encourages women to pay attention to the type and quality of the foods they are consuming, rather than just counting calories or restricting food intake.

The Galveston Diet recommends that women focus on fueling their bodies with nutrient-dense, whole foods, rather than relying on processed or convenience foods that are high in calories but low in nutrition. This means consuming a diet that is high in protein, healthy fats, and fiber, while also being low in sugar, refined carbohydrates, and other unhealthy ingredients.

The Galveston Diet encourages women to eat foods that are high in protein, such as lean meats, fish, poultry, eggs, and plant-based sources of protein, like beans and legumes. Protein is important for maintaining muscle mass and can help to keep women feeling fuller for longer periods of time, which can help with weight management.

Healthy fats are also an important part of Fuel Refocus on the Galveston Diet. Women are encouraged to consume sources of healthy fats like avocados, nuts, seeds, and fatty fish, which can help to reduce inflammation, support brain health, and provide sustained energy throughout the day.

In addition to protein and healthy fats, the Galveston Diet recommends that women consume plenty of fiber-rich foods like fruits, vegetables, and whole grains. Fiber can help to regulate digestion, promote feelings of fullness, and support overall gut health.

By focusing on nutrient-dense, whole foods, rather than just counting calories or restricting food intake, Fuel Refocus on the Galveston Diet aims to help women achieve and maintain a healthy weight, while also improving their overall health and reducing their risk of chronic diseases.

Q&A

CAN I STILL ENJOY MY FAVORITE FOODS ON THE GALVESTON DIET?

Yes, the Galveston diet allows for flexibility and encourages moderation. While it emphasizes whole, unprocessed foods, it also allows for occasional indulgences and encourages mindful eating. The Galveston Diet is not a restrictive diet, and it does not require individuals to completely eliminate their favorite foods. However, the diet does emphasize the importance of choosing nutrient-dense foods that support overall health and well-being.

The Galveston Diet encourages individuals to focus on whole, unprocessed foods, such as fruits, vegetables, lean proteins, and healthy fats. These foods are naturally high in nutrients and can help to reduce inflammation in the body, balance hormones, and support weight loss.

While the Galveston Diet does not require individuals to completely eliminate any specific foods, it does encourage moderation and balance. For example, it may be recommended to limit processed and high-sugar foods, which can contribute to inflammation and weight gain.

In general, the Galveston Diet encourages individuals to make sustainable, long-term changes to their eating habits and lifestyle. This may include incorporating healthier versions of favorite foods or finding ways to enjoy them in moderation while still maintaining overall balance and health.

It is important to note that individual dietary needs and preferences may vary, and it is recommended to speak with a healthcare professional or registered dietitian to create a personalized nutrition plan that meets your individual needs and health goals.
What makes the Galveston Diet different from other diets?
The Galveston Diet is specifically designed for women over 40 and takes into account the hormonal changes that occur during menopause. It focuses on reducing inflammation and balancing hormones to promote weight loss. The Galveston Diet is different from other diets in several ways:

Designed for women over 40: The Galveston Diet was specifically created for women over 40 who are going through menopause. It takes into account the hormonal changes that occur during this time and how they can affect weight loss.

Focus on inflammation and hormones: The Galveston Diet focuses on reducing inflammation in the body and balancing hormones, which can help to promote weight loss and improve overall health. It emphasizes whole, nutrient-dense foods that can help to reduce inflammation, such as fruits, vegetables, lean proteins, and healthy fats.

No calorie counting: Unlike some other diets, the Galveston Diet does not require individuals to count calories or macronutrients. Instead, it focuses on choosing high-quality, nutrient-dense foods that support overall health and well-being.

Emphasis on self-care: The Galveston Diet encourages individuals to focus on self-care and stress management, which can help to support weight loss and overall health. It emphasizes the importance of getting enough sleep, practicing mindfulness, and engaging in regular physical activity.

Support and community: The Galveston Diet offers a supportive community of like-minded individuals who are going through similar experiences. It provides resources and support to help individuals stay motivated and on track with their weight loss and health goals.

IS THE GALVESTON DIET SAFE FOR EVERYONE?

The Galveston Diet is generally considered safe for most people, but it may not be suitable for everyone. It is always recommended to consult with a healthcare professional before starting any new diet or exercise program, especially if you have any medical conditions, allergies, or are taking any medications.

The Galveston Diet may not be appropriate for individuals with certain medical conditions, such as kidney disease or liver disease, as it may place additional stress on these organs. It may also not be suitable for individuals who have a history of disordered eating or have a restrictive relationship with food.

It is important to follow the Galveston Diet as directed and not to restrict calories excessively, as this may lead to nutrient deficiencies and other health problems. It is also important to stay hydrated and to ensure that you are getting all of the necessary vitamins and minerals through your diet or supplementation.

In summary, while the Galveston Diet may be safe and effective for some individuals, it is important to speak with a healthcare professional before starting the program to ensure that it is appropriate for your individual needs and health status.

IS EXERCISE A PART OF THE GALVESTON DIET?

Exercise is a recommended part of the Galveston Diet. The diet emphasizes a holistic approach to weight loss and overall health, which includes regular physical activity. Exercise can help to support weight loss, increase muscle mass, improve cardiovascular health, and boost overall well-being.

The Galveston Diet does not prescribe a specific exercise program or regimen, but rather encourages individuals to find a type of physical activity that they enjoy and can maintain over time. This can include activities such as walking, jogging, cycling, strength training, yoga, or other forms of exercise.

In addition to regular exercise, the Galveston Diet also recommends that individuals focus on getting enough sleep, managing stress, and practicing self-care. These lifestyle factors can have a significant impact on weight loss and overall health, and are an important part of the Galveston Diet approach.

It is important to note that before starting any new exercise program, it is recommended to speak with a healthcare professional to ensure that it is safe and appropriate for your individual needs and health status.

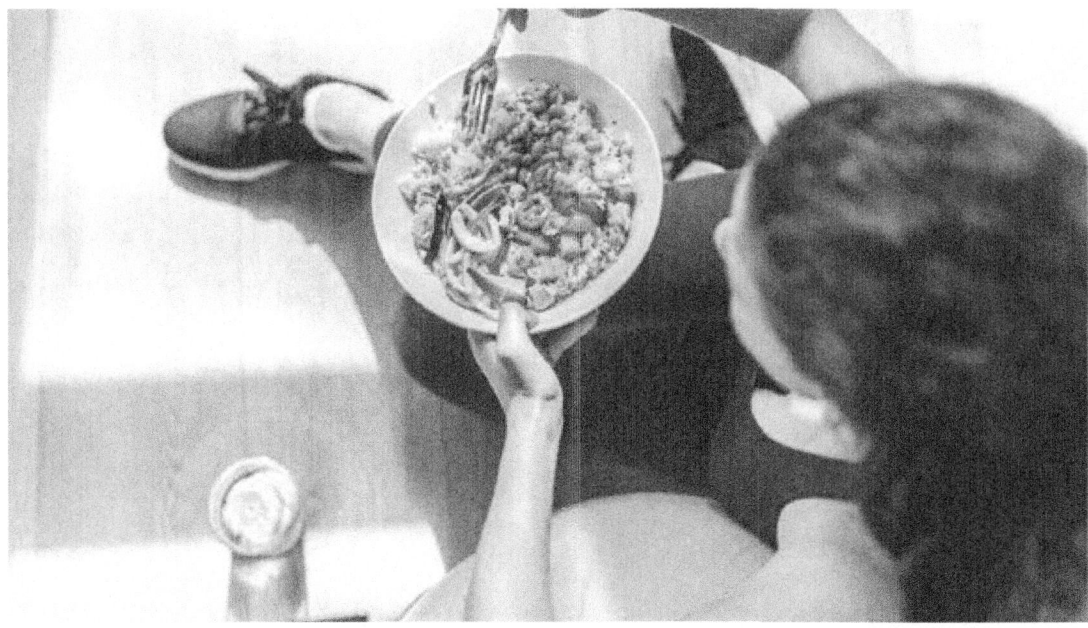

Chapter 4
A Comprehensive Guide to Meal Planning

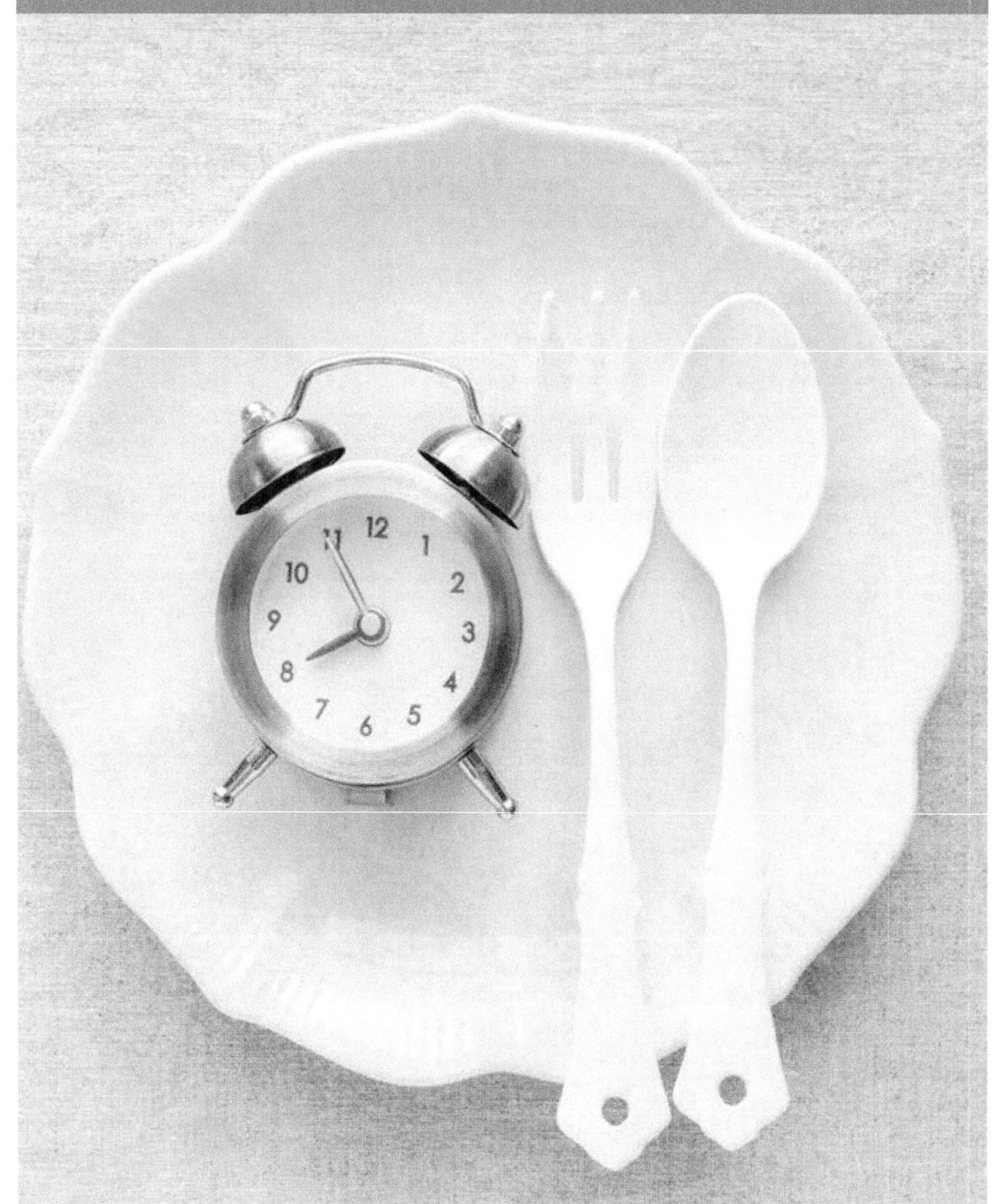

Tips for Planning and Preparing Meals on the Galveston Diet

Planning and preparing meals can be an important aspect of following the Galveston diet. Here are some tips to help you plan and prepare meals on the Galveston diet:

1. Make a grocery list: Before heading to the grocery store, make a list of the foods you need to purchase for the week. This can help you avoid impulse purchases and ensure you have the right foods on hand.
2. Meal prep: Consider prepping your meals in advance to save time during the week. This can include chopping vegetables, cooking proteins, and portioning out meals.
3. Experiment with recipes: Look for recipes that are compatible with the Galveston diet and try out new dishes to keep meals interesting.
4. Batch cook: Consider making larger batches of meals that can be frozen and reheated later in the week. This can help save time and ensure you always have a healthy meal on hand.
5. Use healthy cooking methods: When cooking, use healthy cooking methods such as grilling, baking, or roasting instead of frying or sautéing in unhealthy oils.
6. Pack snacks: Prepare healthy snacks in advance to take with you on the go. This can include items like nuts, seeds, and cut-up vegetables.
7. Use spices and herbs: Experiment with different spices and herbs to add flavor to your meals without adding extra calories or sodium.
8. Consider a meal delivery service: If you don't have the time or energy to prep your meals, consider using a meal delivery service that specializes in the Galveston diet to ensure you are eating the right foods.
9. Stay organized: Keep your pantry and refrigerator organized so you can easily find the foods you need and avoid wasting food.
10. Don't be too strict: While it's important to follow the principles of the Galveston diet, don't be too strict with yourself. Allow for occasional treats and don't be too hard on yourself if you slip up.

Suggestions for Meal Prep and Batch Cooking

Meal prep and batch cooking can be extremely helpful when following the Galveston diet. Here are some suggestions for meal prep and batch cooking:

1. Cook a large batch of protein: Grill or roast a large batch of chicken, turkey, beef, or fish at the beginning of the week. You can then portion out the protein into containers and use it throughout the week for salads, wraps, or stir-fries.
2. Roast vegetables: Roast a large batch of non-starchy vegetables such as broccoli, cauliflower, and Brussels sprouts. These can be used as a side dish or added to salads throughout the week.
3. Make a big salad: Prepare a large salad with mixed greens, vegetables, and protein. Store it in an airtight container and add dressing just before serving.
4. Make a large batch of soup: Soups are a great way to incorporate a variety of vegetables and protein into your meals. Make a large batch of vegetable or chicken soup and store it in individual containers for easy reheating throughout the week.
5. Make a frittata or quiche: A frittata or quiche can be a nutritious and convenient breakfast option. Make a large batch on the weekend and slice it into portions for easy breakfasts throughout the week.
6. Cook grains in advance: If you choose to include grains in your diet, cook a large batch of quinoa, brown rice, or farro at the beginning of the week. Store it in the refrigerator and use it throughout the week for salads or as a side dish.
7. Prep snacks: Cut up vegetables such as carrots, celery, and cucumber and store them in individual containers for easy snacking. You can also portion out nuts, seeds, and dried fruit for a convenient on-the-go snack.

Chapter 5
The Meal Plans and Shopping Lists

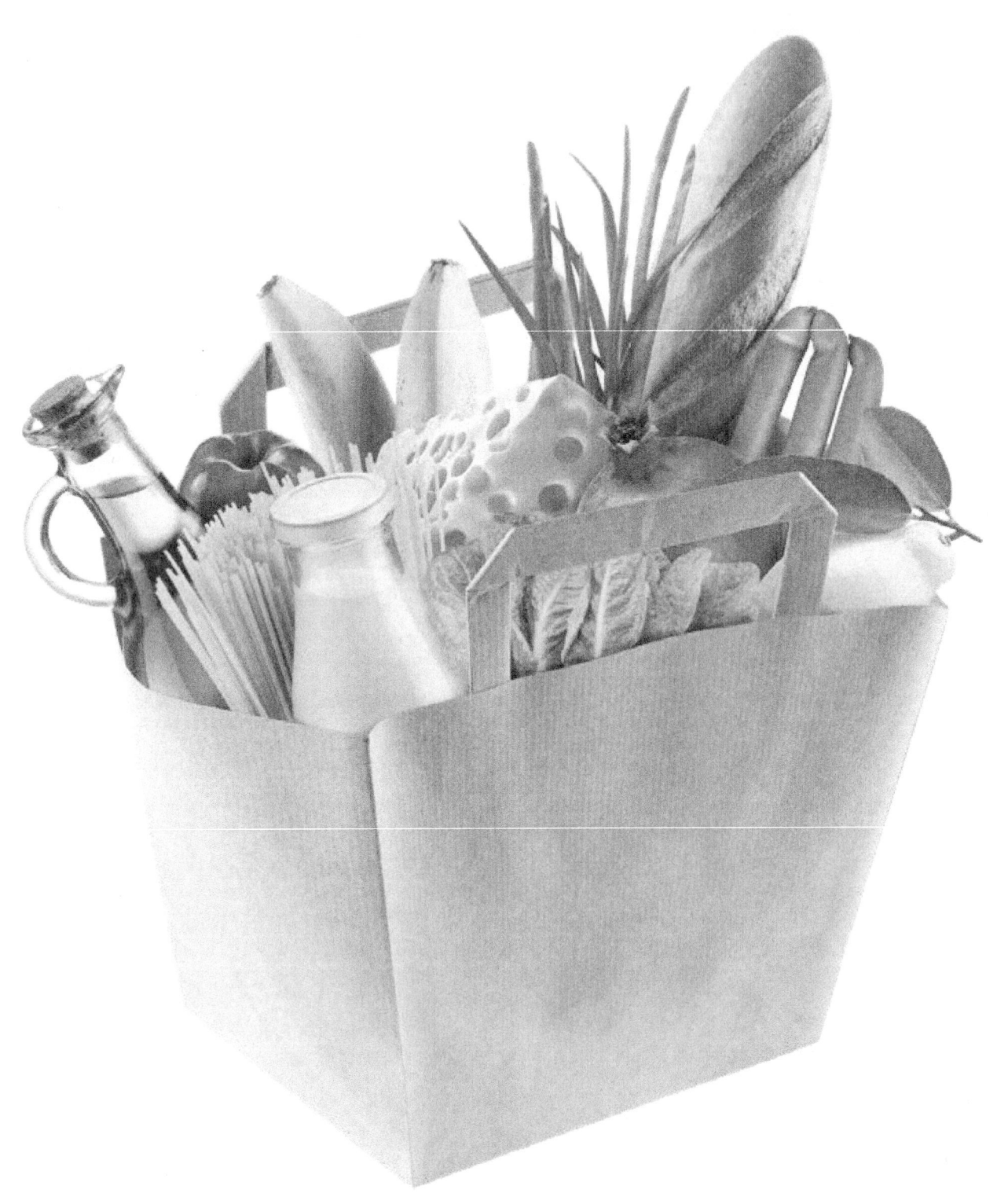

The Conventional Menus: Week 1

Day 1

Meal 1: Olives Fritters
Snack 1: Cheesy Crackers
Meal 2: Lamb-Stuffed Peppers
Snack 2: Cheesy Crackers
Macros: Fat:54, Protein:69, Net Carbs:19, Fiber: 9

Day 2

Meal 1: Olives Fritters
Snack 1: Cheesy Crackers
Meal 2: Lamb-Stuffed Peppers
Snack 2: Cheesy Crackers
Macros: Fat:54, Protein:69, Net Carbs:19, Fiber: 9

Day 3

Meal 1: Olives Fritters
Snack 1: Cheesy Crackers
Meal 2: Lamb-Stuffed Peppers
Snack 2: Cheesy Crackers
Macros: Fat:54, Protein:69, Net Carbs:19, Fiber: 9

Day 4

Meal 1: Olives Fritters
Snack 1: Cheesy Crackers
Meal 2: Lamb-Stuffed Peppers
Snack 2: Cheesy Crackers
Macros: Fat:54, Protein:69, Net Carbs:19, Fiber: 9

Day 5

Meal 1: Olives Fritters
Snack 1: Cheesy Crackers
Meal 2: Lamb-Stuffed Peppers
Snack 2: Cheesy Crackers
Macros: Fat:54, Protein:69, Net Carbs:19, Fiber: 9

Day 6

Meal 1: Mexican Muffins
Snack 1: Cheesy Crackers
Meal 2: Lamb-Stuffed Peppers
Snack 2: Cheesy Crackers
Macros: Fat:57.3, Protein:71.6, Net Carbs:17.7, Fiber: 7

Day 7

Meal 1: Mexican Muffins
Snack 1: Cheesy Crackers
Meal 2: Lamb-Stuffed Peppers
Snack 2: Cheesy Crackers
Macros: Fat:57.3, Protein:71.6, Net Carbs:17.7, Fiber: 7

Shopping List for Week 1

Note: Amounts given here indicate the quantities you need for the week's recipes; they are not always indicative of the quantities in which the items are commonly sold.

Vegetables:
- 3 Zucchinis
- 6 Bell peppers
- 3 Spring onions

Nuts:
- 2 cups Almond flour
- 6 ounces Parmesan cheese

Proteins:
- 1.5 pounds Ground lamb
- 1 cup Ground beef
- 1/2 cup Kalamata olives

Miscellaneous:
- Cooking spray
- 1 Egg
- 2 tablespoons Butter
- 1 teaspoon Keto tomato sauce
- 1 teaspoon Taco seasoning
- 1/4 cup Fresh basil
- 1/2 cup Parsley
- 2 oz Mexican blend cheese

The Conventional Menus: Week 2

Day 1

Meal 1: Salmon & Asparagus Skewers
Snack 1: Herbed Mozzarella Sticks
Meal 2: Chili Eggs
Snack 2: Zucchini Fritters
Macros: Fat: 60.5, Protein: 76.6, Net Carbs: 13.4, Fiber: 4.1

Day 2

Meal 1: Salmon & Asparagus Skewers
Snack 1: Herbed Mozzarella Sticks
Meal 2: Chili Eggs
Snack 2: Zucchini Fritters
Macros: Fat: 60.5, Protein: 76.6, Net Carbs: 13.4, Fiber: 4.1

Day 3

Meal 1: Salmon & Asparagus Skewers
Snack 1: Herbed Mozzarella Sticks
Meal 2: Chili Eggs
Snack 2: Zucchini Fritters
Macros: Fat: 60.5, Protein: 76.6, Net Carbs: 13.4, Fiber: 4.1

Day 4

Meal 1: Salmon & Asparagus Skewers
Snack 1: Herbed Mozzarella Sticks
Meal 2: Chili Eggs
Snack 2: Zucchini Fritters

Macros: Fat: 60.5, Protein: 76.6, Net Carbs: 13.4, Fiber: 4.1

Day 5

Meal 1: Salmon & Asparagus Skewers
Snack 1: Herbed Mozzarella Sticks
Meal 2: Chili Eggs
Snack 2: Zucchini Fritters
Macros: Fat: 60.5, Protein: 76.6, Net Carbs: 13.4, Fiber: 4.1

Day 6

Meal 1: Salmon & Asparagus Skewers
Snack 1: Herbed Mozzarella Sticks
Meal 2: Chili Eggs
Snack 2: Zucchini Fritters
Macros: Fat: 60.5, Protein: 76.6, Net Carbs: 13.4, Fiber: 4.1

Day 7

Meal 1: Salmon & Asparagus Skewers
Snack 1: Herbed Mozzarella Sticks
Meal 2: Chili Eggs
Snack 2: Zucchini Fritters
Macros: Fat: 60.5, Protein: 76.6, Net Carbs: 13.4, Fiber: 4.1

Shopping List for Week 2

Vegetables:
- 1 bunch asparagus
- 2 cups grated zucchini

Fruits:
- 2 lemons

Proteins:
- 1.5 pounds boned skinless salmon, cut into 2-inch chunks
- 8 eggs
- 8 sticks full-fat string cheese, halved horizontally

Nuts:
- ½ cup almond flour
- 2 tablespoons coconut flour
- 1 cup very finely grated Parmesan cheese

Miscellaneous:
- 2 tablespoons ghee, melted
- 1 teaspoon Dijon mustard
- 1 teaspoon garlic powder
- ¼ teaspoon red pepper flakes
- 1 tablespoon Italian seasoning
- ½ teaspoon garlic salt
- ½ cup peanut oil
- 1 teaspoon avocado oil
- ½ cup sour cream
- 2 tablespoons chopped fresh chives

The Conventional Menus: Week 3

Day 1

Meal 1: Lamb Souvlaki
Snack 1: No-Fail Deviled Eggs
Meal 2: Vegetable Low Mein
Snack 2: Creamy Spinach Dip
Macros: Fat:67, Protein:56, Net Carbs:57, Fiber: 16

Day 2

Meal 1: Lamb Souvlaki
Snack 1: No-Fail Deviled Eggs
Meal 2: Vegetable Low Mein
Snack 2: Creamy Spinach Dip
Macros: Fat:67, Protein:56, Net Carbs:57, Fiber: 16

Day 3

Meal 1: Lamb Souvlaki
Snack 1: No-Fail Deviled Eggs
Meal 2: Vegetable Low Mein
Snack 2: Creamy Spinach Dip
Macros: Fat:67, Protein:56, Net Carbs:57, Fiber: 16

Day 4

Meal 1: Lamb Souvlaki
Snack 1: No-Fail Deviled Eggs
Meal 2: Baked Portobello Mushrooms
Snack 2: Creamy Spinach Dip
Macros: Fat:56, Protein:52, Net Carbs:19, Fiber: 14

Day 5

Meal 1: Lamb Souvlaki
Snack 1: No-Fail Deviled Eggs
Meal 2: Baked Portobello Mushrooms
Snack 2: Creamy Spinach Dip
Macros: Fat:56, Protein:52, Net Carbs:19, Fiber: 14

Day 6

Meal 1: Lamb Souvlaki
Snack 1: No-Fail Deviled Eggs
Meal 2: Baked Portobello Mushrooms
Snack 2: Creamy Spinach Dip
Macros: Fat:56, Protein:52, Net Carbs:19, Fiber: 14

Day 7

Meal 1: Lamb Souvlaki
Snack 1: No-Fail Deviled Eggs
Meal 2: Baked Portobello Mushrooms
Snack 2: Creamy Spinach Dip
Macros: Fat:56, Protein:52, Net Carbs:19, Fiber: 14

Shopping List for Week 3

Vegetables:
- 2 medium zucchinis
- 1 red onion
- 1 green bell pepper
- 1 red bell pepper
- 1 white onion
- 1 package frozen spinach
- 2 Portobello mushroom caps

Fruits:
- 1 lemon
- 1 lime
- 1 key lime

Proteins:
- 1 pound lamb shoulder
- 8 hardboiled eggs
- 6 ounces cream cheese
- 8 ounces sour cream

Miscellaneous:
- Olive oil
- Apple cider vinegar
- Dried oregano
- Spelt noodles
- Onion powder
- Sesame oil
- Dijon mustard
- Apple cider vinegar
- Ranch seasoning
- Grated Parmesan cheese
- Alkaline soy sauce

The Conventional Menus: Week 4

Day 1

Meal 1: Swede & Carrot Purée
Snack 1: Baked Olives
Meal 2: Sesame Chicken Stir-Fry
Snack 2: Mushroom Bites
Macros: Fat:58, Protein:46, Net Carbs:32, Fiber: 12

Day 2

Meal 1: Swede & Carrot Purée
Snack 1: Baked Olives
Meal 2: Sesame Chicken Stir-Fry
Snack 2: Mushroom Bites
Macros: Fat:58, Protein:46, Net Carbs:32, Fiber: 12

Day 3

Meal 1: Swede & Carrot Purée
Snack 1: Baked Olives
Meal 2: Sesame Chicken Stir-Fry
Snack 2: Mushroom Bites
Macros: Fat:58, Protein:46, Net Carbs:32, Fiber: 12

Day 4

Meal 1: Swede & Carrot Purée
Snack 1: Baked Olives
Meal 2: Sesame Chicken Stir-Fry
Snack 2: Mushroom Bites
Macros: Fat:58, Protein:46, Net Carbs:32, Fiber: 12

Day 5

Meal 1: Mexican Quinoa
Snack 1: Baked Olives
Meal 2: Sesame Chicken Stir-Fry
Snack 2: Mushroom Bites
Macros: Fat:65, Protein:61, Net Carbs:95, Fiber: 12

Day 6

Meal 1: Mexican Quinoa
Snack 1: Baked Olives
Meal 2: Sesame Chicken Stir-Fry
Snack 2: Mushroom Bites
Macros: Fat:65, Protein:61, Net Carbs:95, Fiber: 12

Day 7

Meal 1: Mexican Quinoa
Snack 1: Baked Olives
Meal 2: Sesame Chicken Stir-Fry
Snack 2: Mushroom Bites
Macros: Fat:65, Protein:61, Net Carbs:95, Fiber: 12

Shopping List for Week 4

Vegetables:
- 1 head of cauliflower
- 4 carrots
- 1/2 swede
- 6 cups kale
- 1 shallot
- 2 cloves garlic
- 1 chili pepper
- 1 jalapeño pepper

Fruits:
- 1/2 lemon
- 1 lime

Proteins:
- 1 pound boneless skinless chicken breasts
- 1 egg

Miscellaneous:
- 14 ounces feta cheese
- 1 cup rinsed quinoa
- 1/4 cup Greek yogurt
- 3 tablespoons extra-virgin olive oil
- 1 and 1/4 cups coconut flour
- 2 tablespoons tahini
- 2 cups chicken broth
- 1/2 cup cilantro
- Salt and black pepper to taste
- Paprika

The Vegetarian Menus: Week 1

Day 1

Meal 1: Thyme Radish Mix
Snack 1: Mediterranean Cucumber Bites
Meal 2: Mixed Vegetable Stir-Fry
Snack 2: Cheesy Cauliflower Breadsticks
Macros: Fat:33.6, Protein:22.7, Net Carbs: 217.5, Fiber: 8.5

Day 2

Meal 1: Thyme Radish Mix
Snack 1: Mediterranean Cucumber Bites
Meal 2: Mixed Vegetable Stir-Fry
Snack 2: Cheesy Cauliflower Breadsticks
Macros: Fat:33.6, Protein:22.7, Net Carbs: 217.5, Fiber: 8.5

Day 3

Meal 1: Thyme Radish Mix
Snack 1: Mediterranean Cucumber Bites
Meal 2: Mixed Vegetable Stir-Fry
Snack 2: Cheesy Cauliflower Breadsticks
Macros: Fat:33.6, Protein:22.7, Net Carbs: 217.5, Fiber: 8.5

Day 4

Meal 1: Thyme Radish Mix
Snack 1: Mediterranean Cucumber Bites
Meal 2: Mixed Vegetable Stir-Fry
Snack 2: Cheesy Cauliflower Breadsticks
Macros: Fat:33.6, Protein:22.7, Net Carbs: 217.5, Fiber: 8.5

Day 5

Meal 1: Spiced Okra Curry
Snack 1: Mediterranean Cucumber Bites
Meal 2: Mixed Vegetable Stir-Fry
Snack 2: Cheesy Cauliflower Breadsticks
Macros: Fat:40.4, Protein:26, Net Carbs:229, Fiber: 12.6

Day 6

Meal 1: Spiced Okra Curry
Snack 1: Mediterranean Cucumber Bites
Meal 2: Mixed Vegetable Stir-Fry
Snack 2: Cheesy Cauliflower Breadsticks
Macros: Fat:40.4, Protein:26, Net Carbs:229, Fiber: 12.6

Day 7

Meal 1: Spiced Okra Curry
Snack 1: Mediterranean Cucumber Bites
Meal 2: Mixed Vegetable Stir-Fry
Snack 2: Cheesy Cauliflower Breadsticks
Macros: Fat:40.4, Protein:26, Net Carbs:229, Fiber: 12.6

Shopping List for Vegetarian Week 1

Vegetables:
- 2 lbs chicken breasts
- 1 head of cauliflower
- 4 bell peppers
- 4 onions
- 2 cups radish
- 2 carrots
- 1 celery stalk
- 2 cups broccoli florets
- 1 cup snow peas
- 2 cucumbers
- 1 1/2 cups okra
- 8 cherry tomatoes

Fruits:
- 1 lime

Nuts:
- 1/2 cup chopped cashews

Proteins:
- 2 lbs chicken breasts

Miscellaneous:
- Low-sodium vegetable broth
- Coconut aminos
- Raw honey
- Arrowroot powder
- Sesame oil
- Cream cheese
- Flat-leaf parsley
- Grated sharp cheddar cheese
- Grated Parmesan cheese
- Ground paprika
- Tomato sauce
- Soft-jelly coconut milk

The Vegetarian Menus: Week 2

Day 1

Meal 1: Peppery Rice Bowl
Snack 1: Caprese Stuffed Avocados
Meal 2: Sage Sweet Potato Wedges
Snack 2: Three-Cheese Stuffed Mushrooms
Macros: Fat:56, Protein:24, Net Carbs:93, Fiber: 16.6

Day 2

Meal 1: Peppery Rice Bowl
Snack 1: Caprese Stuffed Avocados
Meal 2: Sage Sweet Potato Wedges
Snack 2: Three-Cheese Stuffed Mushrooms
Macros: Fat:56, Protein:24, Net Carbs:93, Fiber: 16.6

Day 3

Meal 1: Peppery Rice Bowl
Snack 1: Caprese Stuffed Avocados

Meal 2: Sage Sweet Potato Wedges
Snack 2: Three-Cheese Stuffed Mushrooms
Macros: Fat:56, Protein:24, Net Carbs:93, Fiber: 16.6

Day 4

Meal 1: Peppery Rice Bowl
Snack 1: Caprese Stuffed Avocados
Meal 2: Sage Sweet Potato Wedges
Snack 2: Three-Cheese Stuffed Mushrooms
Macros: Fat:56, Protein:24, Net Carbs:93, Fiber: 16.6

Day 5

Meal 1: Chinese Trail Mix
Snack 1: Caprese Stuffed Avocados
Meal 2: Sage Sweet Potato Wedges
Snack 2: Three-Cheese Stuffed Mushrooms
Macros: Fat:62, Protein:24, Net Carbs:52, Fiber: 16.6

Day 6

Meal 1: Chinese Trail Mix
Snack 1: Caprese Stuffed Avocados
Meal 2: Sage Sweet Potato Wedges
Snack 2: Three-Cheese Stuffed Mushrooms
Macros: Fat:62, Protein:24, Net Carbs:52, Fiber: 16.6

Day 7

Meal 1: Chinese Trail Mix
Snack 1: Caprese Stuffed Avocados
Meal 2: Sage Sweet Potato Wedges
Snack 2: Three-Cheese Stuffed Mushrooms
Macros: Fat:62, Protein:24, Net Carbs:52, Fiber: 16.6

- 1 tablespoon olive oil
- 6 teaspoons spice mix
- ½ tablespoon grapeseed oil
- ¾ cup tomato sauce, alkaline
- ¾ cup vegetable broth, homemade
- 2 tablespoons balsamic vinegar
- Sea salt and pepper to taste
- ½ teaspoon Chinese five-spice powder
- 1 tablespoon extra-virgin olive oil
- ½ cup small mozzarella balls or bocconcini
- ½ cup grated Parmesan cheese
- ½ cup grated Gruyère cheese

Shopping List for Vegetarian Week 2

Vegetables:
- 2 bell peppers (red and green)
- 4 sweet potatoes
- 1 shallot
- 1 medium onion
- 4 garlic cloves
- 3 button mushrooms
- ¼ teaspoon cayenne pepper

Fruits:
- 8 cherry tomatoes
- ½ cup dried blueberries
- 2 avocados

Nuts:
- 1 cup walnuts

Proteins:
- 12 oz boneless skinless chicken breasts
- 4 oz bacon
- 4 oz chorizo sausage
- 6 eggs

Miscellaneous:
- 2 tablespoons pesto
- 2 cups cooked brown rice
- 2 teaspoons low-sodium soy sauce

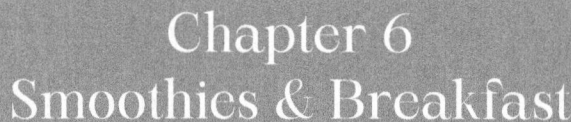

Chapter 6
Smoothies & Breakfast

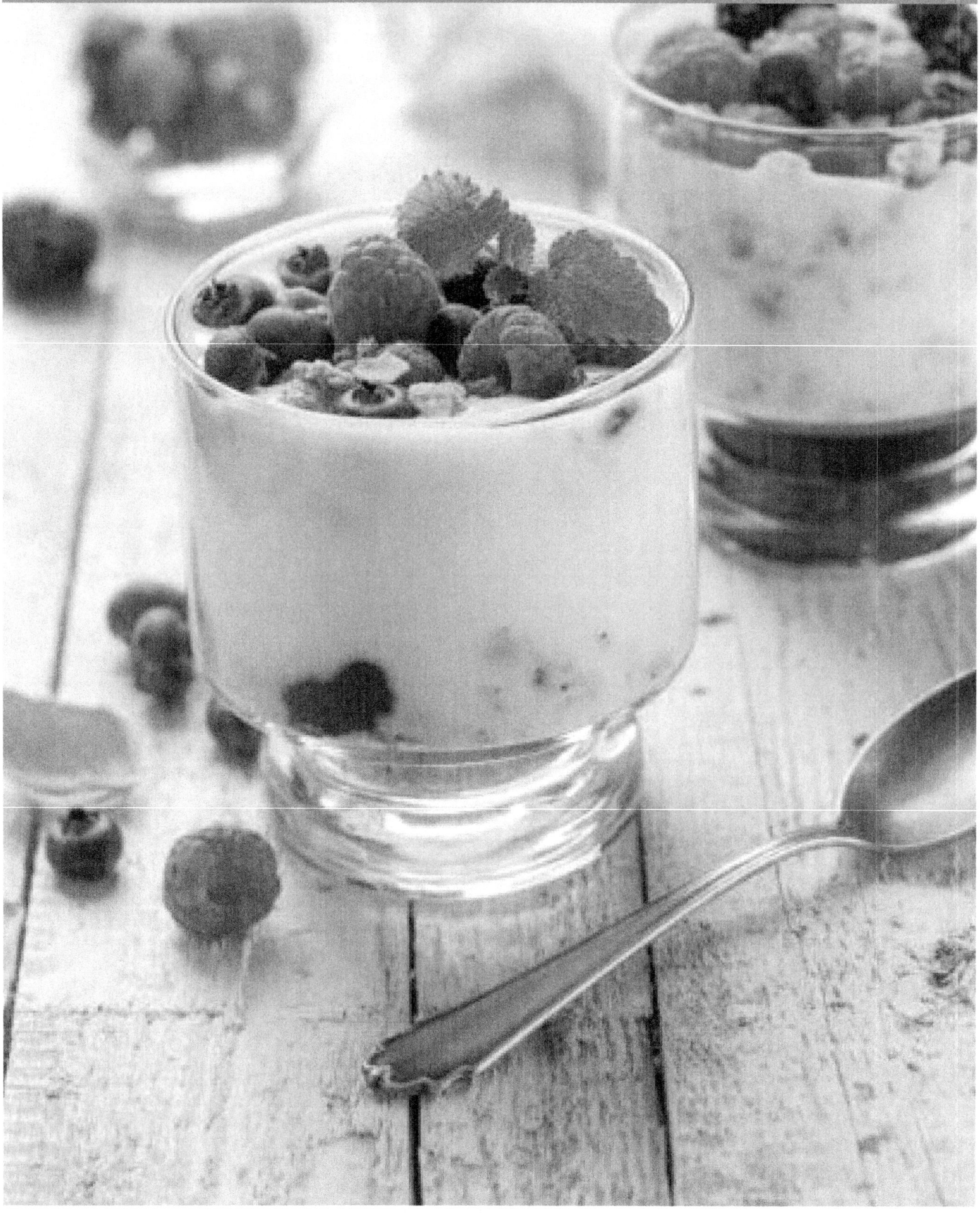

Tropical Papaya Smoothie

Prep time: 5 minutes | Cook time: 5 minutes | Serves 2

- 1 cup soft-jelly coconut milk, unsweetened
- ½ of large papaya, cut into cubes
- 2 Medjool dates, pitted
- 1½ cup frozen mango
- 3 tablespoons grated soft-jelly coconut

1. Place all the ingredients in a blender in the order stated in the ingredients list and then pulse until smooth.
2. Serve immediately.

PER SERVING

Cories:191 | Fat:3.2 g | Protein:12.6 g |Carb:31.5 g |Fiber: 5.8 g

Chai Smoothie

Prep time: 5 minutes | Cooking time: 10 minutes | Serves 2

- 1 cup unsweetened almond milk
- 1 cup pure pumpkin purée
- 1 tablespoon pure maple syrup
- 1 teaspoon grated fresh peeled ginger
- ¼ teaspoon ground cinnamon
- ⅛ teaspoon ground nutmeg
- Pinch ground cloves
- Pinch ground cardamom
- 4 ice cubes

1. In a blender, combine the almond milk, pumpkin, maple syrup, ginger, cinnamon, nutmeg, cloves, and cardamom. Blend until smooth.
2. Add the ice and blend until thick.

PER SERVING

Calories 88| Total fat 2g| Saturated fat 0g| Carbohydrates 18g| Fiber 4g| Protein 2g

Soothing Smoothie

Prep time: 5 minutes | Cook time: 5 minutes | Serves 2

- 2 cups hemp milk
- ½ cup strawberries
- ½ cup blueberries
- ¼ cup sea moss
- 1 cup diced peaches
- 2 Medjool dates, pitted

1. Place all the ingredients in a blender in the order stated in the ingredients list and then pulse until smooth.
2. Serve immediately.

PER SERVING

Cories:360 | Fat:6 g | Protein:11 g |Carb:75 g |Fiber: 18 g

Cleansing Smoothie

Prep time: 5 minutes | Cook time: 5 minutes | Serves 2

- 2 cups walnut milk, unsweetened
- 4 oranges, peeled
- ½ teaspoon cayenne pepper
- 2 cups frozen mango pieces
- 4 tablespoons avocado oil

1. Place all the ingredients in a blender in the order stated in the ingredients list and then pulse until smooth.
2. Serve immediately.

PER SERVING

Cories:330 | Fat:6 g | Protein:10 g |Carb:66 g |Fiber: 6 g

Watermelon Smoothie

Prep time: 5 minutes | Cook time: 5 minutes| Serves2

- 1 cup walnut milk, unsweetened
- 3 cups watermelon chunks
- 2 tablespoons raisins
- 3 tablespoons basil leaves
- 2 Medjool dates, pitted

1. Place all the ingredients in a blender in the order stated in the ingredients list and then pulse until smooth.
2. Serve immediately.

PER SERVING

Cories: 227 | Fat:3.4 g | Protein:8.6 g |Carb:44.2 g |Fiber: 1.8 g

Vegan Rib Roast

Prep time: 5 minutes | Cook time: 15 minutes| Serves 2

- 2 caps of Portobello mushrooms, ½ -inch thick sliced
- 1 teaspoon of sea salt
- ½ cup Alkaline Barbecue Sauce
- 1 teaspoon onion powder
- ¼ cup spring water
- Extra:
- ½ teaspoon cayenne pepper
- 1 tablespoon grapeseed oil

1. Place mushroom slices in a container with a lid, add BBQ sauce, all the seasoning, and water, cover with a lid, and then shake until coated.
2. Place the container into the refrigerator and then let it marinate for a minimum of 6 hours, shaking every 2 hours.
3. When ready to cook, take a griddle pan, place it over medium-high heat, brush with oil and let it preheat.
4. Thread three slices of mushrooms in a skewer, then arrange these skewers on the pan and then cook for 15 minutes, flipping every 3 minutes.
5. Serve straight away.

PER SERVING

Clories:108 |Fats0.6 g |Protein6 g |Carb18 g |Fiber 3 g

Morning Detox Smoothie

Prep time: 5 minutes | Cook time: 5 minutes| Serves2

- 1 cup frozen blueberries
- 1 teaspoon Maca
- 1 cup kale leaves
- ¼ cup sea moss gel
- 1 cup lettuce leaves
- 1 tablespoon Moringa powder
- 1 tablespoon linseeds

1. Place all the ingredients in a blender in the order stated in the ingredients list and then pulse until smooth.
2. Serve immediately.

PER SERVING

Cories:227 | Fat:3.4 g | Protein:8.6 g |Carb:44.2 g |Fiber: 1.8 g

Olives Fritters

Prep time: 5 minutes | Cook time: 12 minutes | Serves 6

- Cooking spray
- ½ cup parsley, chopped
- 1 egg
- ½ cup almond flour
- Salt and black pepper to the taste
- 3 spring onions, chopped
- ½ cup kalamata olives, pitted and minced
- 3 zucchinis, grated

1. In a bowl, mix all the ingredients except the Cooking spray , stir well and shape medium fritters out of this mixture.
2. Place the fritters in your air fryer's basket, grease them with Cooking spray and cook at 380 degrees F for 6 minutes on each side. Serve them as an appetizer.

PER SERVING

Calories 165|Fat 5|Fiber 2|Carbs 3|Protein 7

Mexican Muffins
Prep time: 10 minutes | Cook time: 15 minutes | Serves 4

- 1 cup ground beef
- 1 teaspoon taco seasoning
- 2 oz Mexican blend cheese, shredded
- 1 teaspoon keto tomato sauce
- Cooking spray

1. Preheat the air fryer to 375F. Meanwhile, in the mixing bowl mix up ground beef and taco seasonings. Spray the muffin molds with Cooking spray.
2. Then transfer the ground beef mixture in the muffin molds and top them with cheese and tomato sauce.
3. Transfer the muffin molds in the preheated air fryer and cook them for 15 minutes.

PER SERVING

Calories 123|Fat 8.3|Fiber 0|Carbs 1.7|Protein 9.6

Avocado Smoothie
Prep time: 5 minutes | Cook time: 5 minutes| Serves2

- 3 cups walnut milk, unsweetened
- 2 medium pears, diced
- 2 avocados, peeled, pitted,
- ¼ cup sea moss gel
- 2 teaspoons maca powder

1. Place all the ingredients in a blender in the order stated in the ingredients list and then pulse until smooth.
2. Serve immediately.

PER SERVING

Cories:370 | Fat:21 g | Protein:8 g |Carb:44 g |Fiber: 11 g

Zucchini Hummus Wrap
Prep time: 5 minutes | Cook time: 5 minutes| Serves 2

- ½ cup iceberg lettuce
- 1 zucchini, sliced
- 2 cherry tomatoes, sliced
- 2 spelt flour tortillas
- 4 tablespoons homemade hummus
- ¼ teaspoon salt
- 1/8 teaspoon cayenne pepper
- 1 tablespoon grapeseed oil

1. Take a grill pan, grease it oil and let it preheat over medium-high heat setting.
2. Meanwhile, place zucchini slices in a large bowl, sprinkle with salt and cayenne pepper, drizzle with oil and then toss until coated.
3. Arrange zucchini slices on the grill pan and then cook for 2 to 3 minutes per side until developed grill marks.
4. Assemble tortillas and for this, heat the tortilla on the grill pan until warm and develop grill marks and spread 2 tablespoons of hummus over each tortilla.
5. Distribute grilled zucchini slices over the tortillas, top with lettuce and tomato slices, and then wrap tightly.
6. Serve straight away.

PER SERVING

Clories:264.5 |Fats5.1 g |Protein8.5 g |Carb34.5 g |Fiber 5 g

Paprika Chips
Prep time: 2 minutes | Cook time: 5 minutes | Serves 6

- 8 ounces cheddar cheese, shredded
- 1 teaspoon sweet paprika

1. Divide the cheese in small heaps in a pan that fits the air fryer, sprinkle the paprika on top, introduce the pan in the machine and cook at 400 degrees F for 5 minutes.
2. Cool the chips down and serve them.

PER SERVING

Calories 150|Fat 4|Fiber 3|Carbs 4|Protein 6

Sea moss Banana Smoothie

Prep time: 5 minutes | Cook time: 5 minutes| Serves4

- 2 burro bananas, frozen
- 3 dates, pitted
- 1/8 teaspoon sea salt
- 3 tablespoons sea moss gel
- ¼ cup hemp seeds
- 6 ice cubes
- 2 cups water, chilled

1. Place all the ingredients in a blender in the order stated in the ingredients list and then pulse until smooth.
2. Serve immediately.

PER SERVING

Cories:312.2 | Fat:6.3 g | Protein:6 g |Carb:64 g |Fiber: 11.6 g

Zucchini Crackers

Prep time: 15 minutes | Cook time: 20 minutes | Serves 16

- 1 cup zucchini, grated
- 2 tablespoons flax meal
- 1 teaspoon salt
- 3 tablespoons almond flour
- ¼ teaspoon baking powder
- ¼ teaspoon chili flakes
- 1 tablespoon xanthan gum
- 1 tablespoon butter, softened
- 1 egg, beaten
- Cooking spray

1. Squeeze the zucchini to get rid of vegetable juice and transfer in the big bowl. Add flax meal, salt, almond flour, baking powder, chili flakes, xanthan gum, and stir well. After this, add butter and egg.
2. Knead the non-sticky dough. Place it on the baking paper and cover with the second sheet of baking paper. Roll up the dough into the flat square.
3. After this, remove the baking paper from the dough surface. Cut it on medium size crackers.
4. Line the air fryer basket with baking paper and put the crackers inside in one layer. Spray them with Cooking spray . Cook them at 355F for 20 minutes.

PER SERVING

Calories 46|Fat 3.9|Fiber 1.3|Carbs 2.1|Protein 1.8

Vegan Portobello Burgers

Prep time: 5 minutes | Cook time: 5 minutes| Serves 2

- 2 Portobello mushroom caps
- ½ of avocado, sliced
- 1 cup purslane
- 2 teaspoons dried basil
- 2 tablespoons olive oil
- ¼ teaspoon salt
- 1 teaspoon dried oregano
- ½ teaspoon cayenne pepper

1. Switch on the oven, then set it to 425 degrees F and let it preheat.
2. Prepare the marinade and for this, take a small bowl, pour in oil, add cayenne pepper, onion powder, oregano, and basil and then stir until mixed.
3. Take a cookie sheet, line it with a foil, brush with oil, place mushroom caps on it, evenly pour the marinade over mushroom caps and then let them marinate for 10 minutes.
4. Then bake the mushroom caps for 20 minutes, flipping halfway, until tender and cooked.
5. When done, place mushroom caps on two plates, top the caps with avocado and purslane evenly and then serve.

PER SERVING

Clories:354 |Fats32.8 g |Protein3.7 g |Carb14.4 g |Fiber 4.4 g

Mushroom Steak

Prep time: 5 minutes | Cook time: 15 minutes | Serves 2

- 2 portabella mushroom caps, 1/8-inch thick sliced
- ½ cup sliced green bell peppers
- ½ cup sliced white onions
- ½ cup sliced red bell peppers
- ¼ cup alkaline sauce
- ½ teaspoon of sea salt
- ½ tablespoon onion powder
- ½ teaspoon dried oregano
- ½ teaspoon dried thyme
- ½ tablespoon grapeseed oil
- 2 spelt flatbread, toasted

1. Take a medium bowl, place sauce in it, add all the seasoning, and then whisk until combined.
2. Add mushroom slices, toss until coated, and then let them marinate for a minimum of 30 minutes, tossing halfway.
3. Then take a pan, place it over medium-high heat, add oil and when hot, add onion and pepper and cook for 3 to 5 minutes until tender-crisp.
4. Add mushroom slices, stir until mixed and continue cooking for 5 minutes.
5. Distribute vegetables evenly between flatbread, roll them, and then serve.

PER SERVING

Clories:302 |Fats18 g |Protein2 g |Carb27 g |Fiber 3 g

Chard and Lime Pasta

Prep time: 5 minutes | Cook time: 5 minutes | Serves 2

- 1 head of Swiss chard, cut into ½-inch pieces
- 1 cup spelt pasta, cooked
- 2 green onions, sliced
- ¼ cup cilantro
- 1 key lime, juiced, zested
- ¼ teaspoon salt
- ¼ teaspoon cayenne pepper
- 1 tablespoon olive oil

1. Take a large skillet pan, place it over medium heat, add oil and when hot, add chard pieces and then cook for 4 minutes or more until wilted.
2. Remove pan from heat, transfer chards to a large bowl, add remaining ingredients and then toss until combined.
3. Serve straight away.

PER SERVING

Clories:224 |Fats7 g |Protein7 g |Carb33 g |Fiber 2 g

Spiced Mushroom Bowl

Prep time: 5 minutes | Cook time: 10 minutes | Serves 2

- 1 ½ cup sliced mushrooms
- 8 cherry tomatoes, chopped
- 1 medium onion, peeled, sliced
- ¾ cup vegetable broth, homemade
- 6 teaspoons spice mix
- ¼ teaspoon salt
- ½ tablespoon grapeseed oil
- ¼ teaspoon cayenne pepper
- ¾ cup tomato sauce, alkaline
- 6 tablespoons soft-jelly coconut milk

1. Take a large skillet pan, place it over medium heat, add oil and warm, add onion, and then cook for 5 minutes until golden brown.
2. Add spice mix, add remaining ingredients into the pan except for okra, stir until mixed, and then bring the mixture to a simmer.
3. Add mushrooms, stir until mixed, and then cook for 10 to 15 minutes over medium-low heat setting until cooked.
4. Serve straight away.

PER SERVING

Clories:186 |Fats3.4 g |Protein2.1 g |Carb36.7 g |Fiber 3.5 g

Vegan Veggie Fritters

Prep time: 5 minutes | Cook time: 15 minutes | Serves 2

- 1 cup chickpea flour
- 200g mushrooms, chopped
- 1 medium green bell pepper, cored, chopped
- 1 tablespoon onion powder
- 2 medium white onions, peeled, chopped
- 1 teaspoon of sea salt
- 1 tablespoon oregano
- 1/8 teaspoon cayenne pepper
- 1 tablespoon grapeseed oil
- 1 tablespoon basil leaves, chopped
- ½ cup spring water

1. Take a large bowl, place all the vegetables in it, add all the seasonings, basil and oregano, stir until mixed, and then let the mixture rest for 5 minutes.
2. Add chickpea flour, stir until mixed and then stir in water until well combined and smooth.
3. Take a large skillet pan, place it over medium heat, add oil and when hot, ladle vegetable mixture in it in portions, press down each portion, and then cook for 3 to 4 minutes per side until cooked and golden brown.
4. Serve straight away.

PER SERVING

Clories:281.5 |Fats15.2 g |Protein13.8 g |Carb26.2 g |Fiber 5 g

Chapter 7
Eggs

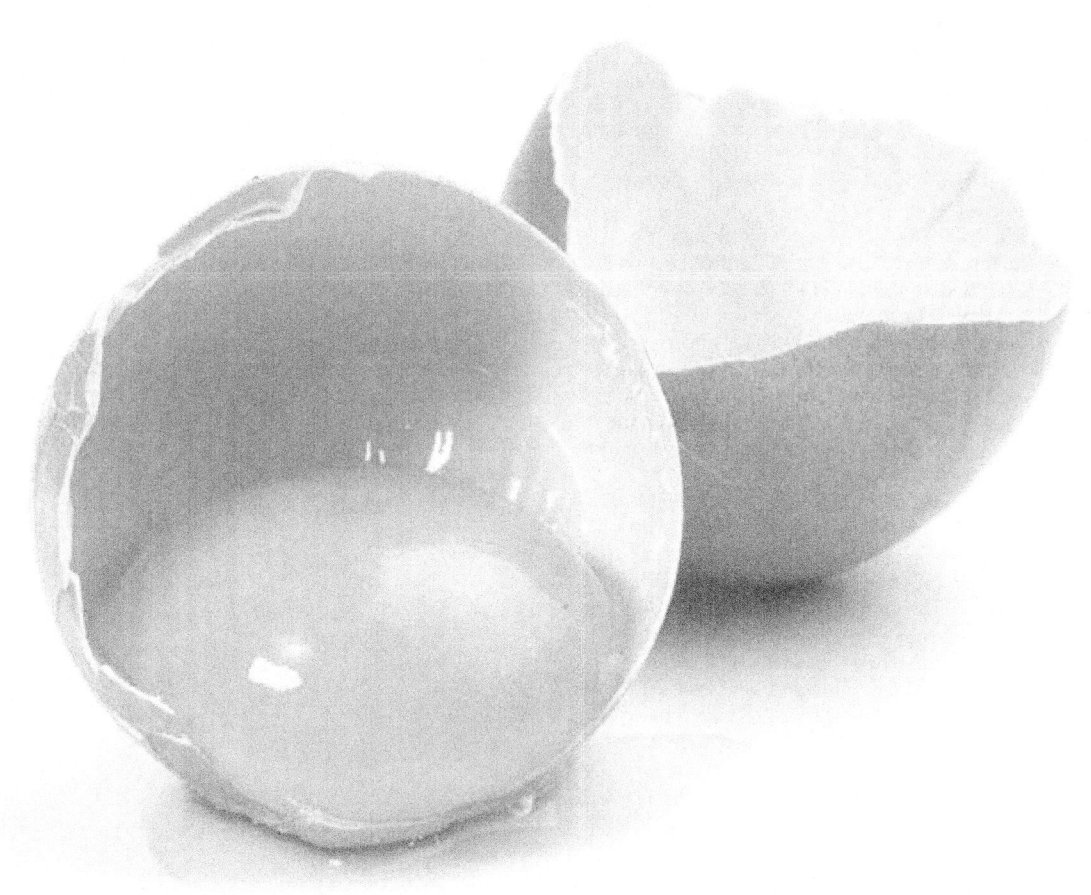

Reuben Egg Rolls
Prep time: 15 minutes | Cook time: 10 minutes | Serves 2

- 1 (8-ounce) package cream cheese, softened
- ½ pound cooked corned beef, chopped
- ½ cup drained and chopped sauerkraut
- ½ cup shredded Swiss cheese (about 2 ounces)
- 20 slices prosciutto
- THOUSAND ISLAND DIPPING SAUCE:
- ¾ cup mayonnaise
- ¼ cup chopped dill pickles
- ¼ cup tomato sauce
- 2 tablespoons Swerve confectioners'-style sweetener or equivalent amount of liquid or powdered sweetener
- ⅛ teaspoon fine sea salt
- Fresh thyme leaves, for garnish
- Ground black pepper, for garnish
- Sauerkraut, for serving (optional)

1. Spray the air fryer basket with avocado oil. Preheat the air fryer to 400°F.
2. Make the filling: Place the cream cheese in a medium-sized bowl and stir to break it up. Add the corned beef, sauerkraut, and Swiss cheese and stir well to combine.
3. Assemble the egg rolls: Lay 1 slice of prosciutto on a sushi mat or a sheet of parchment paper with a short end toward you. Lay another slice of prosciutto on top of it at a right angle, forming a cross. Spoon 3 to 4 tablespoons of the filling into the center of the cross.
4. Fold the sides of the top slice up and over the filling to form the ends of the roll. Tightly roll up the long piece of prosciutto, starting at the edge closest to you, into a tight egg roll shape that overlaps by an inch or so. (Note: If the prosciutto rips, it's okay. It will seal when you fry it.) Repeat with the remaining prosciutto and filling.
5. Place the egg rolls in the air fryer seam side down, leaving space between them. (If you're using a smaller air fryer, cook in batches if necessary.) Cook for 10 minutes, or until the outside is crispy.
6. While the egg rolls are cooking, make the dipping sauce: In a small bowl, combine the mayo, pickles, tomato sauce, sweetener, and salt. Stir well and garnish with thyme and ground black pepper. (The dipping sauce can be made up to 3 days ahead.)
7. Serve the egg rolls with the dipping sauce and sauerkraut if desired. Best served fresh. Store leftovers in an airtight container in the refrigerator for up to 5 days or in the freezer for up to a month. Reheat in a preheated 400°F air fryer for 4 minutes, or until heated through and crispy.

PER SERVING

Calories 321 | Fat 29g | Protein 13g | Total Carbs 1g | Fiber 0.1g

Spinach Eggs
Prep time: 15 minutes | Cook time: 20 minutes | Serves 4

- 1 tablespoon avocado oil
- ½ teaspoon chili flakes
- 6 eggs, beaten
- 2 cups spinach, chopped

1. In the mixing bowl, mix chili flakes with eggs and spinach.
2. Then brush the air fryer mold with avocado oil. Pour the egg mixture inside and transfer the mold in the air fryer.
3. Cook the meal at 365F for 20 minutes.

PER SERVING

Calories 103 | Fat 7.1 | Fiber 0.5 | Carbs 1.3 | Protein 8.8

Paprika Egg Cups
Prep time: 15 minutes | Cook time: 3 minutes | Serves 2

- 2 eggs
- 1 tablespoon cream cheese
- 1 teaspoon smoked paprika

1. Crack the eggs into the ramekins and top them with smoked paprika and cream cheese.
2. Cook the eggs in the air fryer at 400F for 3 minutes.

PER SERVING

Calories 83 | Fat 6.3 | Fiber 0.4 | Carbs 1.1 | Protein 6.1

Basil Scotch Eggs

Prep time: 15 minutes | Cook time: 20 minutes| Serves 4

- 4 medium eggs, hard-boiled, peeled
- 2 cups ground pork
- 1 teaspoon dried basil
- ½ teaspoon salt
- 2 tablespoons almond flour

1. In the mixing bowl, mix ground pork with basil, salt, and almond flour.
2. Then make 4 balls from the meat mixture.
3. Fill every meatball with cooked egg and put it in the air fryer.
4. Cook the meal at 375F for 20 minutes.

PER SERVING

Calories 199|Fat 14|Fiber 0.4|Carbs 1.1|Protein 16.3

Eggs with Peppers

Prep time: 5 minutes | Cook time: 30 minutes| Serves 4

- 2 bell peppers, sliced
- 4 eggs, beaten
- 1 teaspoon avocado oil
- ½ teaspoon white pepper

1. Brush the air fryer basket with avocado oil.
2. Then mix the bell peppers with white pepper and put inside the air fryer basket.
3. Pour the beaten eggs over the bell peppers and bake the meal at 360F for 20 minutes.

PER SERVING

Calories 84|Fat 4.7|Fiber 0.9|Carbs 5.1|Protein 6.2

Chili Eggs

Prep time: 5 minutes | Cook time: 10 minutes| Serves 8

- 8 eggs
- 1 teaspoon chili flakes
- 1 teaspoon avocado oil

1. Brush the air fryer basket with avocado oil and crack the eggs inside.
2. Sprinkle the eggs with chili flakes and bake them at 360F for 10 minutes.

PER SERVING

Calories 64|Fat 4.5|Fiber 0.1|Carbs 0.4|Protein 5.6

Spiced Eggs

Prep time: 10 minutes | Cook time: 20 minutes| Serves 4

- 8 eggs
- 1 teaspoon dried basil
- 1 teaspoon ground black pepper
- 1 teaspoon dried oregano
- 1 teaspoon avocado oil

1. Brush the air fryer basket with avocado oil from inside.
2. Then crack the eggs inside and top them with ground black pepper and dried oregano.
3. Bake the meal at 355F for 20 minutes.

PER SERVING

Calories 130 fat 9|Fiber 0.4|Carbs 1.3|Protein 11.2

Bacon and Eggs Avocado
Prep time: 5 minutes | Cook time: 17 minutes | Serves 4

- 1 large egg
- 1 avocado, halved, peeled, and pitted
- 2 slices bacon
- Fresh parsley, for serving (optional)
- Sea salt flakes, for garnish (optional)

1. Spray the air fryer basket with avocado oil. Preheat the air fryer to 320°F. Fill a small bowl with cool water.
2. Soft-boil the egg: Place the egg in the air fryer basket. Cook for 6 minutes for a soft yolk or 7 minutes for a cooked yolk. Transfer the egg to the bowl of cool water and let sit for 2 minutes. Peel and set aside.
3. Use a spoon to carve out extra space in the center of the avocado halves until the cavities are big enough to fit the soft-boiled egg. Place the soft-boiled egg in the center of one half of the avocado and replace the other half of the avocado on top, so the avocado appears whole on the outside.
4. Starting at one end of the avocado, wrap the bacon around the avocado to completely cover it. Use toothpicks to hold the bacon in place.
5. Place the bacon-wrapped avocado in the air fryer basket and cook for 5 minutes. Flip the avocado over and cook for another 5 minutes, or until the bacon is cooked to your liking. Serve on a bed of fresh parsley, if desired, and sprinkle with salt flakes, if desired.
6. Best served fresh. Store extras in an airtight container in the fridge for up to 4 days. Reheat in a preheated 320°F air fryer for 4 minutes, or until heated through.

PER SERVING

Calories 536 | fat 46g | protein 18g | total carbs 18g | fiber 14g

Bacon and Spinach Egg Muffins
Prep Time: 7 Minutes | Cook Time: 12 To 14 Minutes | Serves 6

- 6 large eggs
- ¼ cup heavy (whipping) cream
- ½ teaspoon sea salt
- ¼ teaspoon freshly ground black pepper
- ¼ teaspoon cayenne pepper (optional)
- ¾ cup frozen chopped spinach, thawed and drained
- 4 strips cooked bacon, crumbled
- 2 ounces shredded Cheddar cheese

1. In a large bowl (with a spout if you have one), whisk together the eggs, heavy cream, salt, black pepper, and cayenne pepper (if using).
2. Divide the spinach and bacon among 6 silicone muffin cups. Place the muffin cups in your air fryer basket.
3. Divide the egg mixture among the muffin cups. Top with the cheese.
4. Set the air fryer to 300°F. Cook for 12 to 14 minutes, until the eggs are set and cooked through.

PER SERVING

Total Calories: 180|Total fat: 14g|Total carbohydrates: 2g|Fiber: 1g|Erythritol: 0g|Net carbs: 1g|Protein: 11g

Cheddar Eggs
Prep time: 5 minutes | Cook time: 30 minutes | Serves 4

- 4 eggs, beaten
- 1 teaspoon avocado oil
- 2 oz Cheddar cheese, shredded

1. Brush the ramekins with avocado oil.
2. Then mix eggs with cheese and pour the mixture inside ramekins.
3. Bake the meal at 355F for 25 minutes.

PER SERVING
Calories 122|Fat 9.2|Fiber 0.1|Carbs 0.6|Protein 9.1

Baked Eggs
Prep time: 10 minutes | Cook time: 10 minutes | Serves 3

- 3 eggs
- ½ teaspoon ground turmeric
- ¼ teaspoon salt
- 3 bacon slices
- 1 teaspoon butter, melted

1. Brush the muffin silicone molds with ½ teaspoon of melted butter. Then arrange the bacon in the silicone molds in the shape of circles. Preheat the air fryer to 400F. Cook the bacon for 7 minutes.
2. After this, brush the center of every bacon circle with remaining butter. Then crack the eggs in every bacon circles, sprinkle with salt and ground turmeric.
3. Cook the bacon cups for 3 minutes more.

PER SERVING
Calories 178|Fat 13.6|Fiber 0.1|Carbs 0.9|Protein 12.6

Classic Egg Sandwich
Prep Time: 10 Minutes | Cook Time: 12 To 14 Minutes | Serves 1

- Avocado oil spray
- 1 large egg
- Sea salt
- Freshly ground black pepper
- 2 tablespoons unsalted butter, at room temperature
- 2 slices keto-friendly bread
- 2 slices Cheddar cheese
- ¼ avocado, sliced
- Hot sauce, for serving

1. Line a small air fryer-safe cake pan with parchment paper. Spray a 3½-inch egg ring with oil, then place it in the prepared pan.
2. Place the pan in the air fryer and set to 300°F. Let preheat for 5 minutes.
3. Once the air fryer is preheated, crack an egg into the egg ring. Season with salt and pepper. Cook for 6 to 8 minutes, until the egg is set. Remove from the pan.
4. Spread the butter on one side of each bread slice and place them in the pan. Cook for 4 minutes, or until the butter is melted and the bread is lightly toasted.
5. Place the egg on one of the toasted bread slices, and top with the cheese slices. Cook until the cheese melts, about 2 minutes.
6. Top with the avocado and hot sauce, place the second bread slice on top, and serve.

Per Serving (With 1 Down Home Biscuit)
Total Calories: 735|Total fat: 66g|Total carbohydrates: 11g|Fiber: 6g|Erythritol: 0g|Net carbs: 5g|Protein: 24g

Spinach and Feta Egg Bake

Prep Time: 7 Minutes | Cook Time: 23 To 25 Minutes | Serves 2

- Avocado oil spray
- ⅓ cup diced red onion
- 1 cup frozen chopped spinach, thawed and drained
- 4 large eggs
- ¼ cup heavy (whipping) cream
- Sea salt
- Freshly ground black pepper
- ¼ teaspoon cayenne pepper
- ½ cup crumbled feta cheese
- ¼ cup shredded Parmesan cheese

1. Spray a deep 7-inch air fryer-safe pan with oil. Put the onion in the pan, and place the pan in the air fryer basket. Set the air fryer to 350°F and cook for 7 minutes.
2. Sprinkle the spinach over the onion.
3. In a medium bowl, beat the eggs, heavy cream, salt, black pepper, and cayenne. Pour this mixture over the vegetables.
4. Top with the feta and Parmesan cheese. Cook for 16 to 18 minutes, until the eggs are set and lightly brown.

PER SERVING

Total Calories: 424|Total fat: 32g|Total carbohydrates: 11g|Fiber: 3g|Erythritol: 0g|Net carbs: 8g|Protein: 26g

---

Meritage Eggs

Prep time: 5 minutes | Cook time: 8 minutes| Serves 2

- 2 teaspoons unsalted butter (or coconut oil for dairy-free), for greasing the ramekins
- 4 large eggs
- ½ teaspoon fine sea salt
- ¼ teaspoon ground black pepper
- 2 tablespoons heavy cream (or unsweetened, unflavored almond milk for dairy-free)
- 3 tablespoons finely grated Parmesan cheese (or Kite Hill brand chive cream cheese style spread, softened, for dairy-free)
- Fresh thyme leaves, for garnish (optional)

1. Preheat the air fryer to 400°F. Grease two 4-ounce ramekins with the butter.
2. Crack 2 eggs into each ramekin and divide the thyme, salt, and pepper between the ramekins. Pour 1 tablespoon of the heavy cream into each ramekin. Sprinkle each ramekin with 1½ tablespoons of the Parmesan cheese.
3. Place the ramekins in the air fryer and cook for 8 minutes for soft-cooked yolks (longer if you desire a harder yolk).
4. Garnish with a sprinkle of ground black pepper and thyme leaves, if desired. Best served fresh.

PER SERVING

Calories 331 | Fat 29g | Protein 16g | Total Carbs 2g | Fiber 0.2g

---

Scotch Eggs

Prep time: 15 minutes | Cook time: 13 minutes | Serves 4

- 4 medium eggs, hard-boiled, peeled
- 9 oz ground beef
- 1 teaspoon garlic powder
- ¼ teaspoon cayenne pepper
- 1 oz coconut flakes
- ¼ teaspoon curry powder
- 1 egg, beaten
- 1 tablespoon almond flour
- Cooking spray

1. In the mixing bowl combine together ground beef and garlic powder. Add cayenne pepper, almond flour, and curry powder. Stir the meat mixture until homogenous. After this, wrap the peeled eggs in the ground beef mixture.
2. In the end, you should get meat balls. Coat every ball in the beaten egg and then sprinkle with coconut flakes. Preheat the air fryer to 400F.
3. Then spray the air fryer basket with Cooking spray and place the meat eggs inside. Cook the eggs for 13 minutes. Carefully flip the scotch eggs on another side after 7 minutes of Cooking.

PER SERVING

Calories 272|Fat 16|Fiber 1.5|Carbs 4.3|Protein 28.6

Chapter 8
Soups & Stews

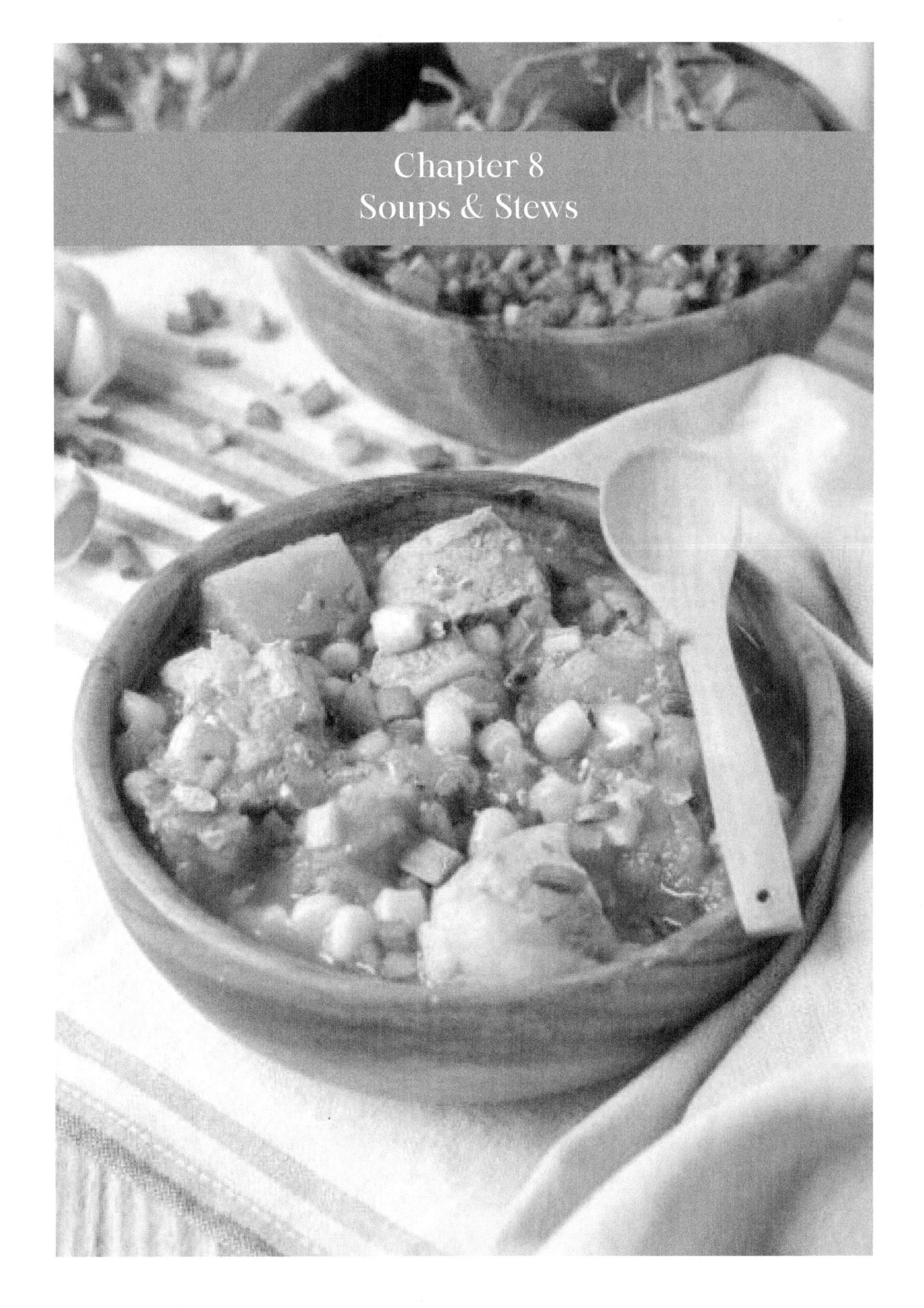

Gut-Healing Bone Broth

Prep time: 15 minutes | Cooking time: 8 to 24 hours | Serves 4

- 2 pounds beef marrow bones
- 4 garlic cloves
- 3 medium carrots, chopped
- 2 celery stalks, chopped
- 1 medium onion, chopped
- 2 bay leaves
- 1 tablespoon apple cider vinegar
- Filtered water, to cover

1. In a 6-quart slow cooker, combine the bones, garlic, carrots, celery, onion, bay leaves, and vinegar.
2. Cover with filtered water. Set the cooker on low and simmer for at least 8 hours and up to 24 hours.
3. Skim off and discard any foam that forms on the surface.
4. Ladle the broth through a fine-mesh sieve or cheesecloth to strain out the solids.
5. Pour into airtight glass containers.
6. The broth can be kept refrigerated for up to 1 week|just reboil it before use. To freeze, allow the broth to completely cool and then fill jars up to 1 inch below the top to allow for expansion, and keep for 4 to 5 months.

PER SERVING

Calories 40| Total Fat 0g| Saturated Fat 0g| Cholesterol 0mg| Carbohydrates 5g| Fiber 0g| Protein 6g

Garlic And Herb Vegetable Broth

Prep time: 5 minutes | Cook time: 5 minutes | Serves 1

- 1 cup hot Vegetable Broth
- 1 tablespoon salted butter
- 1 small clove garlic, peeled
- ¼ teaspoon dried Italian herbs

1. Add all ingredients to a blender and process until smooth.
2. Serve.

PER SERVING

Calories: 119 | Fat: 12g | Protein: 1g | Sodium: 320mg | Fiber: 3g

Mexican Chicken Broth

Prep time: 5 minutes | Cook time: 5 minutes | Serves 1

- 1 cup hot Chicken Bone Broth Base
- 1 tablespoon salted butter
- 1 teaspoon tomato paste
- ¼ teaspoon cumin
- ¼ teaspoon dried oregano
- ¼ teaspoon chili powder
- ⅛ teaspoon ground black pepper

1. Add all ingredients to a blender and process until smooth.
2. Serve.

PER SERVING

Calories: 138 | Fat: 12g | Protein: 5g | Sodium: 372mg | Fiber: 2g

Lemon Pepper Chicken Broth

Prep time: 5 minutes | Cook time: 5 minutes | Serves 1

- 1 cup hot Chicken Bone Broth Base
- 1 tablespoon salted butter
- ½ teaspoon fresh lemon juice
- ⅛ teaspoon ground black pepper

1. Add all ingredients to a blender and process until smooth.
2. Serve.

PER SERVING

Calories: 130 | Fat: 12g | Protein: 5g | Sodium: 349mg | Fiber: 1g

Chayote Mushroom Stew

Prep time: 5 minutes | Cook time: 40 minutes | Serves 2

- 2/3 cup chayote squash cubes
- 1 cups sliced mushrooms
- 1/3 cup diced white onions
- ½ cup chickpea flour
- 1/3 cup vegetable broth, homemade
- 1/3 tablespoon onion powder
- 2/3 teaspoon sea salt
- 2/3 teaspoon dried basil
- 1/3 teaspoon crushed red pepper
- 2 cups spring water
- ½ tablespoon grapeseed oil
- 1/3 cup hemp milk, homemade

1. Take a medium pot, place it over medium-high heat, add oil and when hot, add onion and mushroom, and then cook for 5 minutes.
2. Switch heat to medium level, pour in 1 cup water, milk, and broth, add chayote and all the seasoning, stir until mixed, and then bring it to a simmer, covering the pan with lid.
3. Pour remaining water into a food processor, add chickpea flour, pulse until blended, add to the pot and then stir until mixed.
4. Switch heat to the low level, simmer for 30 minutes, and then serve.

PER SERVING

Clories:173 |Fats9 g |Protein2 g |Carb20 g |Fiber 2 g

Zoodle Vegetable Soup

Prep time: 5 minutes | Cook time: 15 minutes | Serves 2

- ½ of onion, peeled, cubed
- ½ of green bell pepper, chopped
- ½ of zucchini, grated
- 4 ounces sliced mushrooms, chopped
- ½ cup cherry tomatoes
- ¼ cup basil leaves
- 1 pack of spelt noodles, cooked
- ¼ teaspoon salt
- 1/8 teaspoon cayenne pepper
- ½ of key lime, juiced
- 1 tablespoon grapeseed oil
- 2 cups spring water

1. Take a medium saucepan, place it over medium heat, add oil and when hot, add onion and then cook for 3 minutes or more until tender.
2. Add cherry tomatoes, bell pepper, and mushrooms, stir until mixed, and then continue cooking for 3 minutes until soft.
3. Add grated zucchini, season with salt, cayenne pepper, pour in the water, and then bring the mixture to a boil.
4. Then switch heat to the low level, add cooked noodles and then simmer the soup for 5 minutes.
5. When done, ladle soup into two bowls, top with basil leaves, drizzle with lime juice and then serve.

PER SERVING

Clories:265 |Fats2 g |Protein4 g |Carb57 g |Fiber 13.6 g

Thai Chicken Broth

Prep time: 5 minutes | Cook time: 5 minutes | Serves 1

- 1 cup hot Chicken Bone Broth Base
- 1 tablespoon unsalted butter
- 1 small clove garlic, peeled
- ½ teaspoon coconut aminos
- ¼ teaspoon grated fresh ginger
- ⅛ teaspoon fish sauce
- ⅛ teaspoon ground black pepper

1. Add all ingredients to a blender and process until smooth.
2. Serve.

PER SERVING

Calories: 137 | Fat: 12g | Protein: 5g | Sodium: 453mg | Fiber: 1g

Hungarian Beef Bone Broth

Prep time: 5 minutes | Cook time: 5 minutes | Serves 1

- 1 cup hot Beef Bone Broth Base
- 1 tablespoon salted butter
- 1 small clove garlic, peeled
- ½ teaspoon sweet paprika
- ⅛ teaspoon caraway seeds
- ⅛ teaspoon ground black pepper

1. Add all ingredients to a blender and process until smooth.
2. Serve.

PER SERVING

Calories: 172 | Fat: 12g | Protein: 11g | Sodium: 389mg | Fiber: 2g

Miso Chicken Broth

Prep time: 5 minutes | Cook time: 5 minutes | Serves 1

- 1 cup hot Chicken Bone Broth Base
- 1 tablespoon unsalted butter
- 1¼ teaspoons white miso paste
- ⅛ teaspoon ground black pepper

1. Add all ingredients to a blender and process until smooth.
2. Serve.

PER SERVING

Calories: 143 | Fat: 12g | Protein: 5g | Sodium: 545mg | Fiber: 1g

Creamy Squash Soup

Prep time: 5 minutes | Cook time: 25 minutes | Serves 2

- ½ of medium white onion, peeled, cubed
- 2 cups cubed squash
- ¼ cup basil leaves
- ½ cup soft-jelly coconut cream
- 1/8 teaspoon sea salt
- 1/8 teaspoon cayenne pepper
- 1 tablespoon grapeseed oil
- 1 cup vegetable broth, homemade

1. Take a medium saucepan, place it over medium heat, add oil and when hot, add onion, and then cook for 5 minutes or until softened.
2. Add squash, cook for 10 minutes until golden and begin to soften, pour in the vegetable broth, season with salt and pepper and then bring the soup to boil.
3. Switch heat to medium level and then simmer the soup for 10 minutes until squash turns very soft.
4. Remove pan from heat, puree it by using a stick blender until smooth, and then garnish with basil.
5. Serve straight away.

PER SERVING

Clories:183 | Fats 14.4 g | Protein 1.9 g | Carb 13.4 g | Fiber 2.7 g

Chinese Pork Broth

Prep time: 5 minutes | Cook time: 5 minutes | Serves 1

- 1 cup hot Pork Bone Broth Base
- 1 tablespoon unsalted butter
- ½ teaspoon coconut aminos
- ½ teaspoon grated fresh ginger
- ½ teaspoon rice wine vinegar
- ⅛ teaspoon Chinese five spice powder
- ⅛ teaspoon ground black pepper

1. Add all ingredients to a blender and process until smooth.
2. Serve.

PER SERVING

Calories: 150 | Fat: 12g | Protein: 7g | Sodium: 412mg | Fiber: 1g

Italian Tomato And Herb Beef Bone Broth

Prep time: 5 minutes | Cook time: 5 minutes | Serves 1

- 1 cup hot Beef Bone Broth Base
- 1 tablespoon salted butter
- 1 small clove garlic, peeled
- 1 teaspoon tomato paste
- ¼ teaspoon dried Italian herbs

1. Add all ingredients to a blender and process until smooth.
2. Serve.

PER SERVING

Calories: 172 | Fat: 12g | Protein: 11g | Sodium: 388mg | Fiber: 1g

Pho Beef Bone Broth

Prep time: 5 minutes | Cook time: 5 minutes | Serves 1

- 1 cup hot beef bone broth base
- 1 tablespoon unsalted butter
- 1 small clove garlic, peeled
- ½ teaspoon grated fresh ginger
- ½ teaspoon coconut aminos
- ½ teaspoon fresh lime juice
- ⅛ teaspoon fish sauce
- ⅛ teaspoon Chinese five spice powder

1. Add all ingredients to a blender and process until smooth.
2. Serve.

PER SERVING

Calories: 171 | Fat: 12g | Protein: 11g | Sodium: 489mg | Fiber: 1g

Healthy Alkaline Green Soup

Prep time: 5 minutes | Cook time: 15 minutes | Serves 2

- 2 cups leafy greens
- 1 small zucchini, sliced
- 1 small white onion, peeled, sliced
- 1 medium green bell pepper, cored, sliced
- 2 ½ cups spring water
- ¾ teaspoon salt
- ¼ teaspoon cayenne pepper
- 1 teaspoon dried basil

1. Take a medium pot, place it over medium heat, add all the ingredients, stir until mixed, and then cook for 5 to 10 minutes until the vegetables turn tender-crisp.
2. Remove pot from heat, puree the soup by using an immersion blender and then serve.

PER SERVING

Clories:129 |Fats0.2 g |Protein1.1 g |Carb28 g |Fiber 4.5 g

Butternut Pumpkin Soup

Prep time: 5 minutes | Cook time: 15 minutes | Serves 2

- 2 medium butternut squash, peeled, deseeded, chopped
- 1 medium white onion, peeled, chopped
- 2 cups soft-jelly coconut milk
- Extra:
- 2/3 teaspoon sea salt
- 1 cup spring water

1. Take a large saucepan, place it over medium-high heat, pour in water, and then bring it to a boil.
2. Stir in salt, and add vegetables and then cook for 5 to 10 minutes until vegetables turn tender.
3. Remove pan from heat, add milk and then puree by using an immersion blender until smooth.
4. Serve straight away.

PER SERVING

Clories:133.3 |Fats4.8 g |Protein2.1 g |Carb23.6 g |Fiber 1.3 g

Spicy Soursop and Zucchini Soup

Prep time: 5 minutes | Cook time: 45 minutes | Serves 2

- 1 cup chopped kale
- 2 Soursop leaves, rinsed, rip in half
- ½ cup summer squash cubes
- 1 cup chayote squash cubes
- ½ cup zucchini cubes
- ½ cup wild rice
- ½ cup diced white onions
- 1 cup diced green bell peppers
- 2 teaspoons sea salt
- ½ tablespoon basil
- ¼ teaspoon cayenne pepper
- ½ tablespoon oregano
- 6 cups spring water

1. Take a medium pot, place it over medium-high heat, add soursop leaves, pour in 1 ½ cup water, and then boil for 15 minutes, covering the pan with lid.
2. When done, remove eaves from the broth, switch heat to medium level, add remaining ingredients into the pot, stir until mixed, and then cook for 30 minutes or more until done.
3. Serve straight away.

PER SERVING

Clories:224 |Fats5 g |Protein5.8 g |Carb38.1 g |Fiber 3.4 g

Zoodle Chickpea Soup

Prep time: 5 minutes | **Cook time:** 25 minutes | **Serves 2**

- ½ cup cooked, chickpeas
- ½ of a medium white onion, peeled, diced
- ½ of a large zucchini, chopped
- 1 cup kale leaves
- 1 cup squash cubes
- ¾ teaspoon salt
- ¾ tablespoon chopped thyme, fresh
- ¾ tablespoon tarragon, fresh
- 2 cups vegetable broth, homemade
- 1 ½ cup spring water

1. Take a saucepan, place it over medium-high heat, pour in the ¼ cup broth, add zucchini, onion, and thyme and then cook for 4 minutes.
2. Pour in remaining broth and water, bring it to a boil, switch heat to the low level, and then simmer for 10 to 15 minutes until tender.
3. Add remaining ingredients, stir until mixed, and then continue cooking for 10 minutes or more until cooked.
4. Serve straight away.

PER SERVING

Clories:184.5 |Fats0.3 g |Protein6.8 g |Carb31 g |Fiber 6 g

Kamut Squash Soup

Prep time: 5 minutes | **Cook time:** 35 minutes | **Serves 2**

- 6 tablespoons Kamut berries
- 1 cup chopped white onion
- ½ cup chopped squash
- ½ cup cooked chickpeas
- 1 cup vegetable broth, homemade
- ¼ teaspoon cayenne pepper
- ½ tablespoon chopped tarragon
- 1 bay leaf
- 1 teaspoon chopped thyme
- 1 tablespoon olive oil
- 1 cup spring water, boiling

1. Place Kamut in a small bowl, pour in the boiling water, and let it stand for 30 minutes.
2. Then take a medium pot, place it over medium heat, add oil and when hot, add onion, stir in thyme and tarragon and then cook for 5 minutes until tender.
3. Drain Kamut, add to the pot, add bay leaves, pour in the vegetable broth, and then bring it to boil.
4. Cover the pot with its lid, simmer for 20 to 30 minutes, then stir in cayenne pepper and cook for 5 minutes.
5. Remove bay leaf, add chickpeas, and then cook for 2 minutes.
6. Serve straight away.

PER SERVING

Clories:348.8 |Fats8.8 g |Protein11.3 g |Carb57.2 g |Fiber 7.8 g

Chapter 9
Salads & Sides

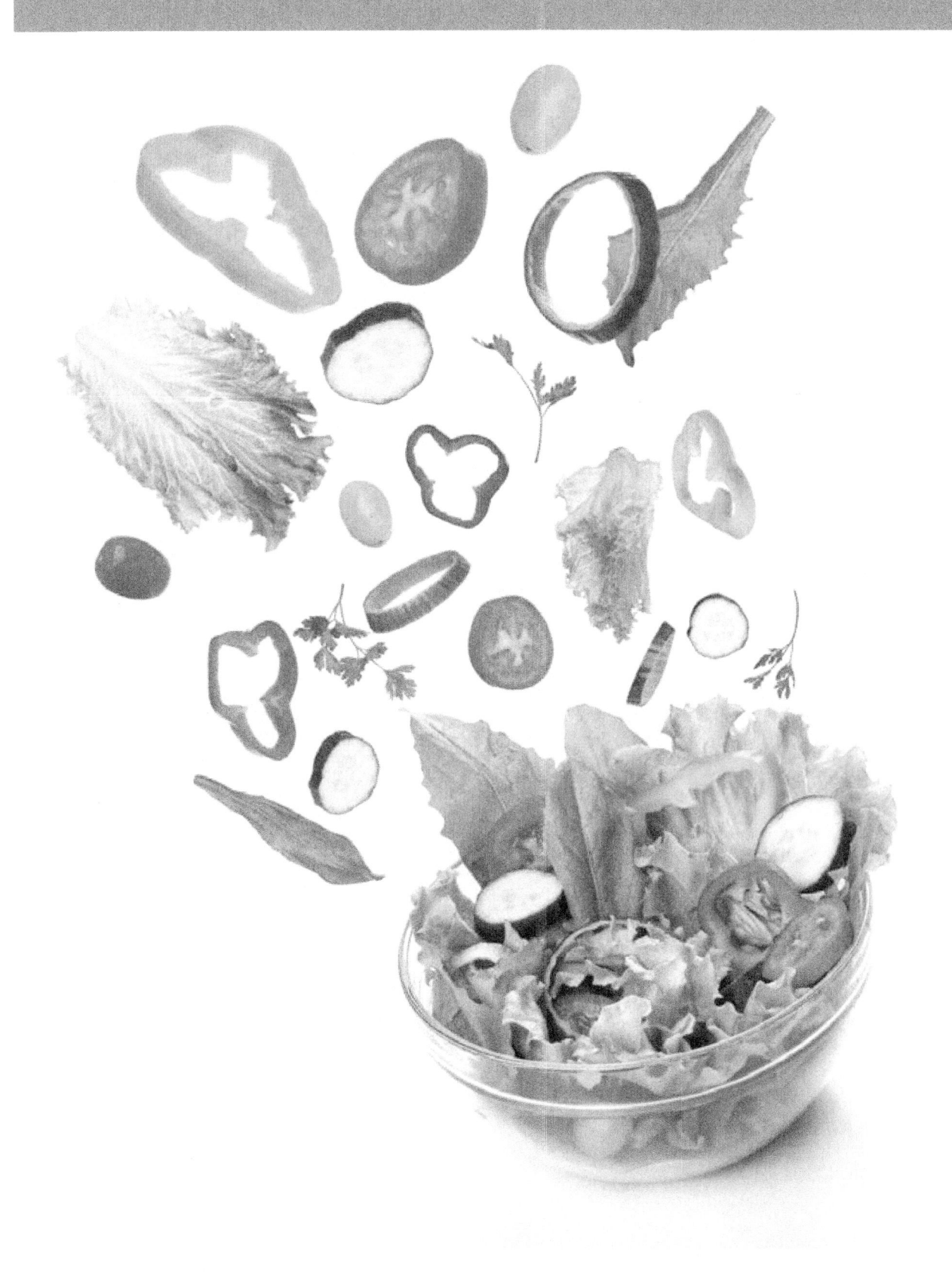

Zesty Citrus Salad

Prep time: 5 minutes | Cook time: 5 minutes | Serves 2

- 4 slices of onion
- ½ of avocado, peeled, pitted, sliced
- 4 ounces arugula
- 1 orange, zested, peeled, sliced
- 1 teaspoon agave syrup
- 1/8 teaspoon salt
- 1/8 teaspoon cayenne pepper
- 2 tablespoons key lime juice
- 2 tablespoons olive oil

1. Distribute avocado, oranges, onion, and arugula between two plates.
2. Mix together oil, salt, cayenne pepper, agave syrup and lime juice in a small bowl and then stir until mixed.
3. Drizzle the dressing over the salad and then serve.

PER SERVING

Clories:265 |Fats24 g |Protein3.8 g |Carb11.6 g |Fiber 6.4 g

Kale and Sprouts Salad

Prep time: 5 minutes | Cook time: 5 minutes | Serves 2

- 2 cups kale leaves
- 1 cup sprouts
- 1 cup cherry tomato
- ½ of avocado, peeled, pitted, diced
- 1 key lime, juiced
- 1 teaspoon agave syrup
- ½ tablespoon olive oil
- 1/8 teaspoon cayenne pepper

1. Take a small bowl, place lime juice in it, add oil and agave syrup and then stir until mixed.
2. Take a salad bowl, place remaining ingredients in it, drizzle with the lime juice mixture and then toss until mixed.
3. Serve straight away.

PER SERVING

Clories:179.2 |Fats14.1 g |Protein3.7 g |Carb13.5 g |Fiber 6.1 g Fiber;

Crunchy Zucchini Fries

Prep time: 15 minutes | Cook time: 30 minutes | Serves 2

- ½ tsp chili powder
- 1 zucchini, cut into strips
- ½ cup almond flour
- Sea salt and pepper to taste
- ½ tsp garlic powder
- 1 tbsp avocado oil

1. Preheat your oven to 425°F. In a bowl, mix the almond flour, chili, powder, salt, garlic powder, and pepper.
2. Brush the zucchini strips with the avocado oil, and roll in the almond flour mixture until well coated. Evenly space the fries on a parchment-lined baking pan. Bake for 20 minutes or until crispy. Serve and enjoy!

PER SERVING

Cal 235| Fat 20g| Carbs 7g| Protein 5g|Fiber 8 g

Massaged Kale Salad

Prep time: 15 minutes|Cooking time:10 minutes|Serves 4

- 2 bunches Lacinato kale, stemmed and torn into bite-size pieces
- 3 scallions, sliced
- 1 avocado, diced
- ¼ cup shelled sunflower seeds
- 2 tablespoons freshly squeezed lemon juice
- 3 tablespoons extra-virgin olive oil
- ½ teaspoon salt
- Freshly ground black pepper
- ¼ cup pomegranate seeds

1. In a large bowl, combine the kale, scallions, avocado, sunflower seeds, lemon juice, olive oil, and salt, and season with pepper.
2. With your hands, massage the salad ingredients for about 5 minutes until the kale begins to soften and the avocado is creamed into the other ingredients.
3. Mix the pomegranate seeds into the salad and serve immediately.

PER SERVING

Calories 249| Total Fat 21g| Saturated Fat 3g| Cholesterol 0mg| Carbohydrates 14g| Fiber 6g| Protein 6g

Peppery Rice Bowl

Prep time: 15 minutes | Cook time: 30 minutes | Serves 4

- 1 shallot, chopped
- 2 cups cooked brown rice
- 2 tbsp extra-virgin olive oil
- 1 red bell pepper, chopped
- 1 green bell pepper, chopped
- 2 tsp low-sodium soy sauce

1. Warm the olive oil in a large nonstick skillet over medium heat. Add the red and green bell peppers and shallot. Cook for about 7 minutes, stirring frequently, until the vegetables start to brown.
2. Add the rice and the soy sauce. Cook for about 3 minutes, stirring constantly, until the rice warms through. Serve and enjoy!

PER SERVING

Cal 265| Fat 9g| Carbs 45g| Protein 4g|Fiber 3

Ginger Stir-Fried Pepper & Broccoli

Prep time: 5 minutes | Cook time: 20 minutes | Serves 4

- 4 cups broccoli florets
- 1 red pepper, cut into strips
- 2 tbsp extra-virgin olive oil
- 1 tbsp grated fresh ginger
- ¼ tsp sea salt
- 2 garlic cloves, minced

1. Warm the olive oil in a large nonstick skillet over medium heat. Add the broccoli, pepper, ginger, and salt. Cook for 5-7 minutes, stirring frequently, until the broccoli begins to brown.
2. Add the garlic. Cook for 30 seconds, stirring constantly. Stir in the sesame seeds. Serve and enjoy!

PER SERVING

Cal 135| Fat 10g| Carbs 9g| Protein 3g|Fiber 4 g

Spicy Sweet Potato Chips

Prep time: 15 minutes | Cook time: 35 minutes | Serves 4

- 2 sweet potatoes, cut into thin strips
- 1 tbsp extra-virgin olive oil
- 1 tsp ground coriander
- ½ tsp black pepper
- ½ tsp paprika
- ¼ tsp cayenne pepper

1. Preheat your oven to 375°F. Arrange the sweet potato strips on a baking sheet into a thin layer.
2. Drizzle with some olive oil. Sprinkle the rest of the ingredients over the top. Toss together gently to evenly and fully coat the potatoes. Bake for around 30 minutes. Serve and enjoy!

PER SERVING

Cal 180| Fat 7g| Carbs 26g| Protein 3g|Fiber 6 g

Cinnamon & Ginger Apple Sautée

Prep time: 15 minutes | Cook time: 20 minutes | Serves 4

- 3 apples, peeled and sliced
- 2 tbsp coconut oil
- 1 tbsp grated ginger
- 1 tsp ground cinnamon
- 1 tbsp raw honey
- A pinch of sea salt

1. Warm the coconut oil in a large nonstick skillet over medium heat.
2. Add the apples, ginger, cinnamon, honey, and salt. Cook for 7-10 minutes, stirring occasionally, until the apples are soft. Serve and enjoy!

PER SERVING

Cal 150| Fat 6g| Carbs 24g| Protein 1g|Fiber 3 g

Basil and Avocado Salad

Prep time: 5 minutes | **Cook time:** 5 minutes | **Serves 2**

- ½ cup avocado, peeled, pitted, chopped
- ½ cup basil leaves
- ½ cup cherry tomatoes
- 2 cups cooked spelt noodles
- 1 teaspoon agave syrup
- 1 tablespoon key lime juice
- 2 tablespoons olive oil

1. Take a large bowl, place pasta in it, add tomato, avocado, and basil in it and then stir until mixed.
2. Take a small bowl, add agave syrup and salt in it, pour in lime juice and olive oil, and then whisk until combined.
3. Pour lime juice mixture over pasta, toss until combined, and then serve.

PER SERVING

Clories:387 |Fats16.6 g |Protein9.4 g |Carb54.3 g |Fiber 8.6 g

Swede & Carrot Purée

Prep time: 15 minutes | **Cook time:** 30 minutes | **Serves 4**

- ½ lemon, zested
- 3 garlic cloves, chopped
- 4 carrots, chopped
- ½ swede, chopped
- ¼ cup chopped thyme
- 1 tbsp extra-virgin olive oil
- Black pepper to taste
- 1 tbsp Greek yogurt

1. Place the carrots, swede, and garlic in a large pan of salted water, bring to the boil, and cook for 12 minutes. Drain.
2. Add the thyme, lemon zest, and olive oil and season with pepper and mash with a potato masher. Stir in a dollop of low-fat Greek yogurt if desired. Serve and enjoy!

PER SERVING

Cal 80| Fat 3g| Carbs 10g| Protein 3g|Fiber 3 g

Delicious Chickpea & Mushroom Bowl

Prep time: 5 minutes | **Cook time:** 15 minutes | **Serves 2**

- 1 ½ cup cooked chickpeas
- 2 zucchinis, spiralized
- 4 small oyster mushrooms, destemmed, diced
- ¼ of white onion, peeled, chopped
- ¼ of red bell pepper, cored, chopped
- 1/3 teaspoon sea salt; 1 teaspoon dried basil
- ¼ teaspoon cayenne pepper; 1 teaspoon dried oregano
- 1 tablespoon grapeseed oil
- 2 ½ cups vegetable broth, homemade

1. Take a medium pot, place it over medium-high heat, add oil and when hot, add red pepper, onion, and mushrooms, season with salt and cayenne pepper, and then cook for 5 minutes until tender.
2. Switch heat to medium-low level, add remaining ingredients except for zucchini noodles, stir until mixed, and then simmer the soup for 15 to 20 minutes.
3. Then add zucchini noodles into the pan, stir until mixed, and then cook for 1 minute or more until thoroughly warmed. Serve straight away.

PER SERVING

Clories:242 |Fats9 g |Protein10 g |Carb34 g |Fiber 9 g

Catalan Spinach

Prep time: 15 minutes | **Cook time:** 20 minutes | **Serves 4**

- 4 cups baby spinach
- 2 garlic cloves, minced
- 2 tbsp extra-virgin olive oil
- 2 tbsp pine nuts
- 1 tbsp raisins
- Sea salt and pepper to taste

1. Warm the olive oil in a large nonstick skillet over medium heat. Add the spinach and cook for 3 minutes, stirring occasionally.
2. Add the garlic. Cook for 30 seconds, stirring constantly. Add the remaining ingredients and cook for about 2 minutes, stirring constantly. Serve and enjoy!

PER SERVING

Cal 82| Fat 7g| Carbs 4g| Protein 1g|Fiber 3 g

Sage Sweet Potato Wedges

Prep time: 15 minutes | Cook time: 30 minutes| Serves 8

- 4 sweet potatoes, cubed
- 4 tbsp extra-virgin olive oil
- 2 tbsp chopped sage
- Sea salt and pepper to taste
- 4 garlic cloves, minced

1. Warm the olive oil in a large nonstick skillet over medium heat.
2. Add the sweet potatoes, sage, and salt. Cook for 10-15 minutes, stirring occasionally, until the sweet potatoes begin to brown. Add the garlic and pepper. Cook for 30 seconds, stirring constantly. Serve and enjoy!

PER SERVING

Cal 200| Fat 6g| Carbs 33g| Protein 2g|Fiber 2 g

Chinese Trail Mix

Prep time: 15 minutes | Cook time: 10 minutes| Serves 4

- ½ tsp Chinese five-spice powder
- ½ cup dried blueberries
- 1 tbsp extra-virgin olive oil
- 1 cup walnuts
- Sea salt to taste

1. Warm the olive oil in a large nonstick skillet over medium heat.
2. Add the walnuts, salt, and Chinese five-spice and cook for 2 minutes, stirring constantly. Remove from the heat and cool. Stir in the blueberries. Serve and enjoy!

PER SERVING

Cal 180| Fat 15g| Carbs 8g| Protein 4g|Fiber 3 g

Mexican Quinoa

Prep time: 15 minutes | Cook time: 35 minutes| Serves 4

- 1 shallot, chopped
- 2 cloves garlic, minced
- 1 tsp olive oil
- 1 can diced tomatoes
- 1 chili pepper, diced
- 1 cup rinsed quinoa
- 1 lime, juiced
- 1 tbsp paprika
- 2 cups chicken broth
- 1 jalapeño pepper, chopped
- ½ cup cilantro

1. Warm the olive oil in a large nonstick skillet over medium heat. Cook the quinoa and shallot in the oil until the onion becomes translucent, about 5 minutes.
2. Add the garlic and pepper and then cook for 4-5 minutes until the garlic is fragrant. Pour in the undrained can of tomatoes with paprika and chicken broth. Allow to simmer for 15-20 minutes until the liquid reduces. Stir in cilantro. Serve.

PER SERVING

Cal 450| Fat 10g| Carbs 73g| Protein 18g|Fiber 3 g

Root-Veggie Chips

Prep time: 15 minutes | Cook time: 50 minutes | Serves 8

- 1 shallot, chopped
- 1 clove garlic, minced
- 1 rutabaga, finely sliced
- 1 turnip, peeled and sliced
- 1 tbsp extra-virgin olive oil
- Sea salt and pepper to taste
- 1 tsp oregano
- 1 tsp paprika

1. Preheat your oven to 375°F. Add shallot, garlic, turnip, and rutabaga to a greased baking dish and spread them into a thin layer.
2. Dust over herbs and spices with a drizzle of olive oil. Bake for 40-50 minutes. Serve.

PER SERVING

Cal 100| Fat 5g| Carbs 15g| Protein 3g|Fiber 5 g

Grilled Romaine Lettuce Salad

Prep time: 5 minutes | Cook time: 5 minutes | Serves 2

- 2 small heads of romaine lettuce, cut in half
- 1 tablespoon chopped basil
- 1 tablespoon chopped red onion
- ¼ teaspoon onion powder
- ½ tablespoon agave syrup
- ½ teaspoon salt
- ¼ teaspoon cayenne pepper
- 2 tablespoons olive oil
- 1 tablespoon key lime juice

1. Take a large skillet pan, place it over medium heat and when warmed, arrange lettuce heads in it, cut-side down, and then cook for 4 to 5 minutes per side until golden brown on both sides.
2. When done, transfer lettuce heads to a plate and then let them cool for 5 minutes.
3. Meanwhile, prepare the dressing and for this, place remaining ingredients in a small bowl and then stir until combined.
4. Drizzle the dressing over lettuce heads and then serve.

PER SERVING

Clories:130 |Fats2 g |Protein2 g |Carb24 g |Fiber 4 g

Chapter 10
Vegan & Vegetarian

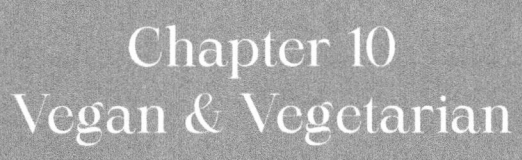

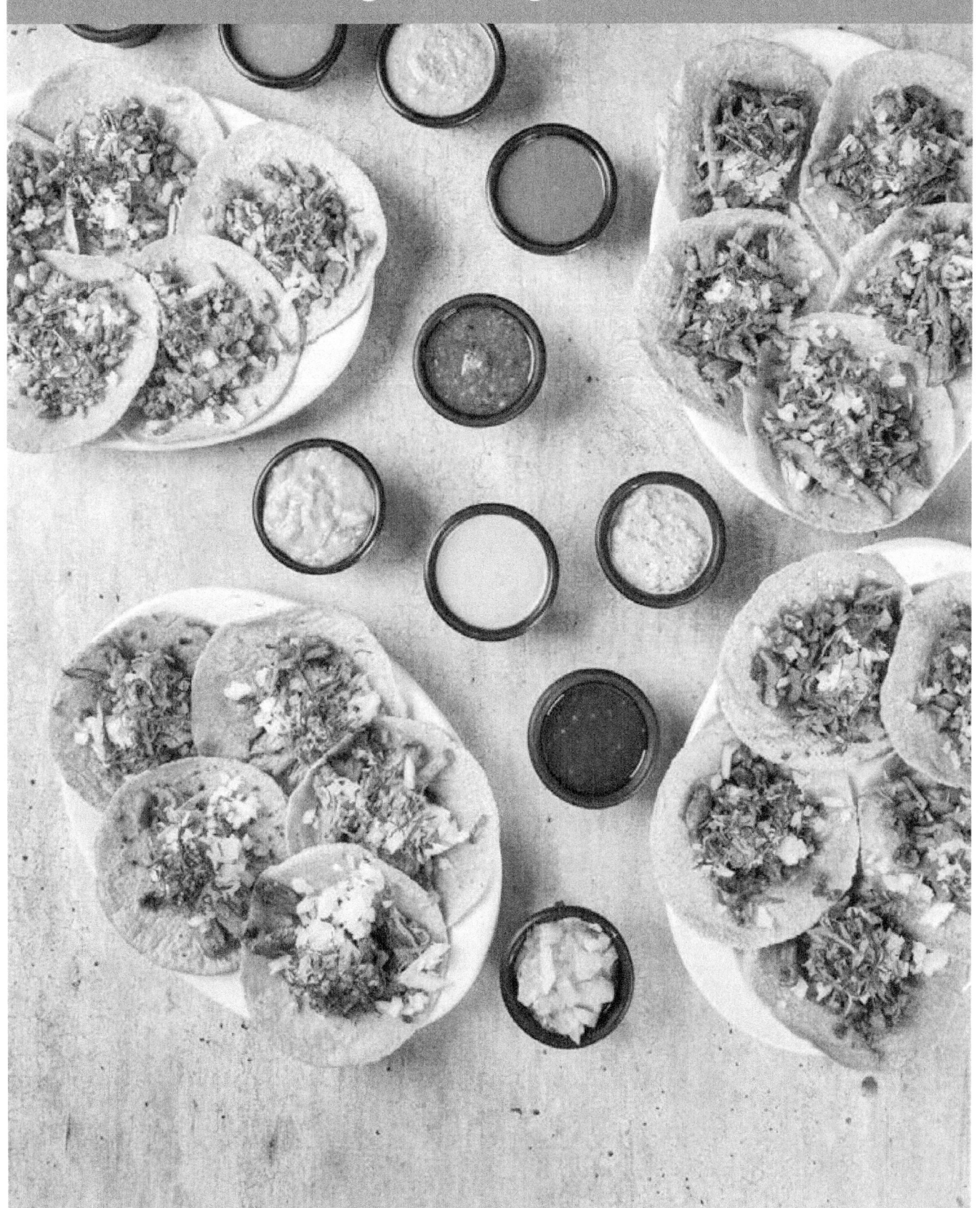

Mixed Vegetable Stir-Fry
Prep time: 30 minutes|Cooking time:11 minutes|Serves 8

- ¼ cup low-sodium vegetable broth
- 1 tablespoon coconut aminos
- 2 teaspoons raw honey
- 1 teaspoon grated fresh ginger
- 1 teaspoon bottled minced garlic
- 1 teaspoon arrowroot powder
- 1½ teaspoons sesame oil
- 1 cup sliced mushrooms
- 2 carrots, thinly sliced, or about 1 to 1½ cups precut packaged carrots
- 2 cups broccoli florets
- 1 cup cauliflower florets
- 1 cup snow peas, halved
- 1 cup bean sprouts
- ¼ cup chopped cashews
- 1 scallion, white and green parts, chopped

1. In a small bowl, whisk the vegetable broth, coconut aminos, honey, ginger, garlic, and arrowroot powder until well combined. Set it aside.
2. In a large skillet or wok over medium-high heat, heat the sesame oil.
3. Add the mushrooms, carrots, and celery. Sauté for 4 minutes.
4. Stir in the broccoli, cauliflower, and snow peas. Sauté for about 4 minutes until crisp-tender.
5. Add the bean sprouts and sauté for 1 minute.
6. Move the vegetables to one side of the skillet and add the sauce. Cook for about 2 minutes, stirring until the sauce has thickened. Stir the vegetables into the sauce, stirring to coat.
7. Serve topped with the cashews and scallion.

PER SERVING
Calories 154| Total fat 6g| Saturated fat 1g| Carbohydrates 21g| Fiber 4g| Protein 7g

Cucumber and Basil Gazpacho
Prep time: 5 minutes | Cook time: 5 minutes| Serves 2

- 1 avocado, peeled, pitted, cold
- 1 cucumber, deseeded, unpeeled, cold
- ½ cup basil leaves, cold
- ½ of key lime, juiced
- 2 cups spring water, chilled
- 1½ teaspoon sea salt

1. Place all the ingredients into the jar of a high-speed food processor or blender and then pulse until smooth.
2. Tip the soup into a medium bowl and then chill for a minimum of 1 hour.
3. Divide the soup evenly between two bowls, top with some more basil and then serve.

PER SERVING
Clories:190 |Fats15 g |Protein4 g |Carb15 g |Fiber 6 g

Vegetable Low Mein
Prep time: 5 minutes | Cook time: 15 minutes| Serves 3

- 2 cups cooked spelt noodles
- ½ of medium green bell pepper, cored, sliced
- ½ of medium red bell pepper, cored, sliced
- 1 medium white onion, cored, sliced
- ½ cup sliced mushrooms
- 2/3 teaspoon salt
- ¼ teaspoon onion powder
- 1/3 teaspoon cayenne pepper
- 1 key lime juiced
- 1 tablespoon sesame oil

1. Take a large skillet pan, place it over medium heat, add oil and when hot, add all the vegetables and cook for 3 to 5 minutes until tender-crisp.
2. Add all the spices, drizzle with lime juice, stir until mixed, and then cook for 1 minute.
3. Add noodles, toss until well mixed and then cook for 2 to 3 minutes until hot.
4. Serve straight away.

PER SERVING
Clories:330 |Fats11 g |Protein10 g |Carb48 g |Fiber 4 g

Snap Peas Mash
Prep time: 15 minutes | Cook time: 6 minutes| Serves 4

- 1 cup snap peas, frozen
- 2 oz Provolone, shredded
- ½ teaspoon chili powder
- ¼ cup chicken stock

1. Mix snap peas with coconut oil and chicken stock and put in the air fryer.
2. Cook them for 6 minutes at 400F.
3. After this, transfer the snap peas in the blender, add all remaining ingredients and blend until smooth.

PER SERVING
Calories 90|Fat 5.2|Fiber 2|Carbs 5.8|Protein 5.7

Prosciutto Asparagus Mix
Prep time: 5 minutes | Cook time: 10 minutes| Serves 4

- 2-pounds asparagus, trimmed
- 2 tablespoons avocado oil
- 1 cup Mozzarella cheese, shredded
- 2 oz prosciutto, chopped

1. Mix asparagus with avocado oil and put it in the air fryer.
2. Then top the vegetables with mozzarella and prosciutto.
3. Cook the meal at 400F for 10 minutes.

PER SERVING
Calories 95|Fat 3.2|Fiber 5.1|Carbs 9.|Protein 10.1

Thyme Radish Mix

Prep time: 10 minutes | **Cook time:** 5 minutes | **Serves 4**

- 2 cups radish, trimmed
- ½ teaspoon onion powder
- ½ teaspoon salt
- ½ teaspoon thyme
- ½ teaspoon ground black pepper
- ½ teaspoon ground paprika
- 1 teaspoon ghee

1. Chop the radish roughly and mix it up with onion powder, salt, thyme, ground black pepper, ad paprika. After this, preheat the air fryer to 375F.
2. Put the roughly chopped radish in the air fryer and cook it for 2 minutes.
3. Then add ghee, shake well and cook the vegetables for 3 minutes more.

PER SERVING

Calories 29|Fat 1.6|Fiber 1.5|Carbs 3.5|Protein 0.7

Veggie Lettuce Wraps

Prep time: 5 minutes | **Cook time:** 5 minutes | **Serves 2**

- ½ cup cherry tomatoes, halved
- 1 avocado, peeled, pitted, sliced
- ½ cup sprouts
- ½ of medium white onion, peeled, sliced
- 2 large lettuce leaves
- 2 tablespoons key lime juice
- ½ tablespoon raisins
- ¼ teaspoon salt
- 1/8 teaspoon cayenne pepper

1. Take a small bowl, add lime juice, add salt and pepper and then stir until mixed.
2. Take a medium bowl, place all the vegetables in it except for lettuce, drizzle with the lime juice mixture and then toss until mixed.
3. Place a lettuce leaves on a plate, top with half of the vegetable mixture, and then roll it tightly.
4. Repeat with the other lettuce wrap and then serve.

PER SERVING

Clories:155 |Fats10.5 g |Protein4.8 g |Carb13.2 g |Fiber 3.5 g Fiber;

Zucchini Linguine

Prep time: 5 minutes | **Cook time:** 10 minutes | **Serves 2**

- 2 zucchini, spiralized
- ½ cup sliced mushrooms
- ½ teaspoon dried thyme
- ½ cup alkaline Avocado sauce
- ¼ cup chopped cilantro
- 1/3 teaspoon salt
- 1/8 teaspoon cayenne pepper
- 1 tablespoon grapeseed oil
- ½ teaspoon dried oregano

1. Take a skillet pan, place it over medium heat, add oil and when hot, add mushrooms and cilantro and then cook for 3 to 5 minutes until tender.
2. Add avocado sauce, season with salt, pepper, oregano, and thyme, stir until mixed and cook for 1 to 2 minutes until warmed.
3. Place zucchini noodles in a large bowl, drizzle with some oil, and then toss until well coated.
4. Add avocado mixture, toss until combined, and then serve.

PER SERVING

Clories:284 |Fats23.6 g |Protein5.7 g |Carb18.8 g |Fiber 9.7 g

Garlic Fennel Bulb

Prep time: 15 minutes | **Cook time:** 15 minutes | **Serves 2**

- 10 oz fennel bulb
- 1 teaspoon avocado oil
- 1 teaspoon garlic powder

1. Chop the fennel bulb roughly and sprinkle with avocado oil and garlic powder.
2. Put the fennel bulb in the air fryer and cook at 375F for 15 minutes.

PER SERVING

Calories 52|Fat 0.6|Fiber 4.6|Carbs 11.5|Protein 2

Paprika Asparagus

Prep time: 5 minutes | **Cook time:** 10 minutes | **Serves 4**

- 1 pound asparagus, trimmed
- 3 tablespoons olive oil
- A pinch of salt and black pepper
- 1 tablespoon sweet paprika

1. In a bowl, mix the asparagus with the rest of the ingredients and toss. Put the asparagus in your air fryer's basket and cook at 400 degrees F for 10 minutes.
2. Divide between plates and serve.

PER SERVING

Calories 200|Fat 5|Fiber 2|Carbs 4|Protein 6

Power Pesto Zoodles

Prep time: 5 minutes | Cook time: 5 minutes | Serves 2

- 2 zucchini
- 1 avocado, peeled, pitted
- ½ cup cherry tomatoes
- 2 tablespoons walnuts
- ½ of key lime, juiced
- ¼ teaspoon salt
- 1/8 teaspoon cayenne pepper
- 2 teaspoons grapeseed oil

1. Prepare the zucchini noodles and for this, cut them into thin strips by using a vegetable peeler or use a spiralizer.
2. Then take a medium skillet pan, add oil in it and when hot, add zucchini noodles in it and then cook for 3 to 5 minutes until tender-crisp.
3. Meanwhile, place the remaining ingredients in a food processor and then pulse until the creamy paste comes together.
4. When zucchini noodles have sautéed, drain and place them in a large bowl and add the blended sauce in it.
5. Add 2 tablespoons of water and then toss until well combined.
6. Garnish the zoodles with grated coconut and then serve.

PER SERVING

Clories:214 |Fats1017.10 g |Protein4.8 g |Carb13.2 g |Fiber 6.1 g

Roasted Squash and Apples

Prep time: 5 minutes | Cook time: 35 minutes | Serves 2

- 1 ½ pounds butternut squash, peeled, deseeded, cut into chunks
- 2 apples, cored, cut into ½-inch pieces
- 2 tablespoons agave syrup
- 1/2 teaspoon sea salt
- 2 tablespoons grapeseed oil

1. Switch on the oven, then set it to 375 degrees F and let it preheat.
2. Meanwhile, take a baking sheet and then spread squash pieces on it.
3. Take a small bowl, pour in oil, stir in salt and allspice until mixed, and then drizzle over squash pieces.
4. Cover the pan with foil and then bake for 20 minutes.
5. Meanwhile, place apple pieces in a medium bowl, drizzle with agave syrup, and then toss until coated.
6. When squash has baked, unwrap the baking sheet, spoon into the bowl containing apple and then stir until mixed.
7. Spread apple-squash mixture evenly on the baking sheet and then continue baking for 15 minutes.
8. Serve straight away.

PER SERVING

Clories:126.4 |Fats4.9 g |Protein1.1 g |Carb22.2 g |Fiber 5.1 g

Mushroom Gravy

Prep time: 5 minutes | Cook time: 15 minutes | Serves 4

- ¾ tablespoon spelt flour
- ¼ of onion, peeled, diced
- 4 ounces sliced mushrooms
- ½ cup walnut milk, homemade
- 1 tablespoon chopped walnuts
- ¼ teaspoon salt
- 1/8 teaspoon cayenne pepper
- ½ teaspoon dried thyme
- 1 tablespoon grapeseed oil
- ¼ cup vegetable broth, homemade

1. Take a medium skillet pan, place it over medium heat, add oil and when hot, add onion and mushrooms, season with 1/16 teaspoon each of salt and cayenne pepper, and then cook for 4 minutes until tender.
2. Stir in spelt flour until coated, cook for 1 minute, slowly whisk in milk and vegetable broth and then season with remaining salt and cayenne pepper.
3. Switch heat to low-level, cook for 5 to 7 minutes until sauce has thickened slightly and then stir in walnuts and thyme.
4. Serve straight away with spelt flour bread.

PER SERVING

Clories:65.3 |Fats1.6 g |Protein3.5 g |Carb9.6 g |Fiber 1 g

Chickpea and Kale Curry

Prep time: 5 minutes | Cook time: 10 minutes | Serves 2

- 2 cups cooked chickpeas
- 2/3 teaspoon salt
- 1 cup Kale leaves
- 2/3 cup soft-jelly coconut cream
- 2 tablespoons grapeseed oil
- 1/3 teaspoon cayenne pepper

1. Switch on the oven, then set it to 425 degrees F and let it preheat.
2. Then take a medium baking sheet, spread chickpeas on it, drizzle with 1 tablespoon oil, sprinkle with all the seasonings and then bake for 15 minutes until roasted.
3. Then take a frying pan, place it over medium heat, add remaining oil and when hot, add kale and cook for 5 minutes.
4. Add roasted chickpeas, pour in the cream, stir until mixed and then simmer for 4 minutes, squashing chickpeas slightly.
5. Serve straight away.

PER SERVING

Clories:522 |Fats38 g |Protein15 g |Carb26 g |Fiber 8 g

Baked Portobello Mushrooms

Prep time: 5 minutes | Cook time: 30 minutes| Serves 4

- 2 caps of Portobello mushrooms, destemmed
- 2/3 teaspoon minced onion
- 2/3 teaspoon minced sage
- 2/3 teaspoon thyme
- 2/3 tablespoon key lime juice
- 2 tablespoons alkaline soy sauce

1. Switch on the oven, then set it to 400 degrees F and let it preheat.
2. Take a baking dish and then arrange mushroom caps in it, cut side up.
3. Take a small bowl, place remaining ingredients in it, stir until mixed, brush the mixture over inside and outside mushrooms, and then let them marinate for 15 minutes.
4. Bake the mushrooms for 30 minutes, flipping halfway, and then serve.

PER SERVING

Clories:72 |Fats2 g |Protein6 g |Carb10 g |Fiber 2 g

Nori Burritos

Prep time: 5 minutes | Cook time: 5 minutes| Serves 2

- 1 avocado, peeled, sliced
- 1 cucumber, deseeded, cut into round slices
- 1 zucchini, sliced
- 2 teaspoons sprouted hemp seeds
- 2 nori sheets
- 1 tablespoon tahini butter
- 2 teaspoons sesame seeds

1. Working on one nori sheet at a time, place it on a cutting board shiny-side-down and then arrange half of each avocado, cucumber and zucchini slices and tahini on it, leaving 1-inch wide spice to the right.
2. Then start folding the sheet over the fillings from the edge that is closest to you, cut into thick slices, and then sprinkle with 1 teaspoon of sesame seeds.
3. Repeat with the remaining nori sheet, and then serve.

PER SERVING

Clories:90 |Fats1.5 g |Protein1.5 g |Carb12.5 g |Fiber 1 g

Chickpea and Mushroom Curry

Prep time: 5 minutes | Cook time: 15 minutes| Serves 2

- 1 cup cooked chickpea
- 1 small white onion, peeled, diced
- ½ of medium green bell pepper, cored, chopped
- 1 cup diced mushrooms
- 8 cherry tomatoes, chopped
- ½ teaspoon salt
- ¼ teaspoon cayenne pepper
- 1 teaspoon grapeseed oil

1. Take a medium skillet pan, place it over medium heat, add oil and when hot, add onion, tomatoes, and bell pepper and then cook for 2 minutes.
2. Add chickpeas and mushrooms, season with and cayenne pepper, stir until combined, and switch heat to medium-low level and then simmer for 10 minutes until cooked, covering the pan with its lid.
3. Serve straight away.

PER SERVING

Clories:194.7 |Fats8.5 g |Protein5.8 g |Carb25.7 g |Fiber 5.4 g

Spiced Okra Curry

Prep time: 5 minutes | Cook time: 15 minutes| Serves 4

- 1 ½ cup okra
- 8 cherry tomatoes, chopped
- 1 medium onion, peeled, sliced
- ¾ cup vegetable broth, homemade
- 6 teaspoons spice mix
- ¼ teaspoon salt
- ½ tablespoon grapeseed oil
- ¼ teaspoon cayenne pepper
- ¾ cup tomato sauce, alkaline
- 6 tablespoons soft-jelly coconut milk

1. Take a large skillet pan, place it over medium heat, add oil and warm, add onion, and then cook for 5 minutes until golden brown.
2. Add spice mix, add remaining ingredients into the pan except for okra, stir until mixed, and then bring the mixture to a simmer.
3. Add okra, stir until mixed, and then cook for 10 to 15 minutes over medium-low heat setting until cooked.
4. Serve straight away.

PER SERVING

Clories:137 |Fats8.4 g |Protein4 g |Carb15 g |Fiber 5.6 g

Chapter 11
Seafood Dishes

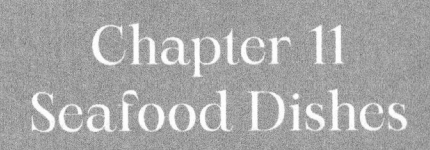

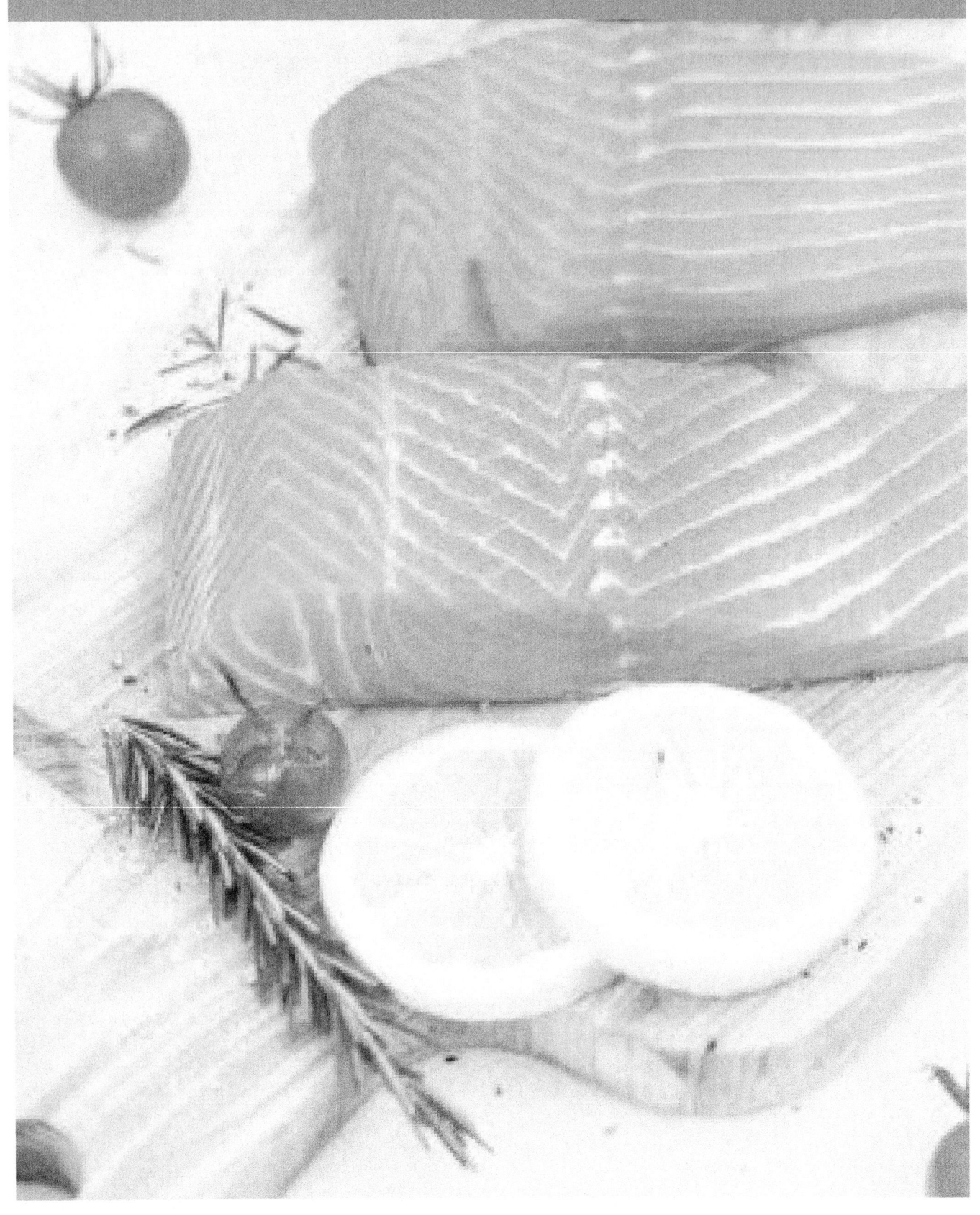

Tilapia Fish Tacos With Cilantro Lime Crema

Prep time: 15 minutes | Cooking time: 8 minutes | Serves 4

- For the cilantro-lime crema
- ½ cup plain whole-milk Greek yogurt
- 2 tablespoons freshly squeezed lime juice
- 1 tablespoon minced fresh cilantro leaves
- ¼ teaspoon garlic powder
- Dash salt
- For the fish tacos
- 8 small corn tortillas
- 1 teaspoon paprika
- ½ teaspoon salt
- ½ teaspoon garlic powder
- ½ teaspoon ground cumin
- ¼ teaspoon cayenne pepper
- 1 pound tilapia fillets
- 2 tablespoons avocado oil
- 1 large avocado, sliced

TO MAKE THE CILANTRO-LIME CREMA

1. In a small bowl, whisk the yogurt, lime juice, cilantro, garlic powder, and salt.
2. Cover and chill until ready to serve.

TO MAKE THE FISH TACOS

1. Preheat the oven to 350°F.
2. Wrap the tortillas in aluminum foil and place them in the oven to warm for about 15 minutes.
3. Meanwhile, in a small bowl, mix the paprika, salt, garlic powder, cumin, and cayenne pepper.
4. Put the fish fillets on a plate, and sprinkle them with the seasoning mixture.
5. In a large skillet over medium-high heat, heat the avocado oil.
6. Add the fish fillets to the skillet. Cook for 3 minutes per side, or until flaky.
7. Lay the warm tortillas out on a work surface. Divide the fish among the tortillas.
8. Serve the fish tacos with the sliced avocado and cilantro-lime crema.

PER SERVING

Calories 363| Total Fat 17g| Saturated Fat 3g| Cholesterol 62mg| Carbohydrates 25g| Fiber 6g| Protein 27g

Whitefish With Spice Rub

Prep time: 5 minutes | Cook time: 15 minutes | Serves 4

- 2 tablespoons Slow-Cooker Ghee, melted, divided
- 4 (6-ounce) whitefish fillets
- 1 tablespoon paprika
- 2 teaspoons ground cumin
- 2 teaspoons onion powder
- 2 teaspoons salt
- 1 teaspoon ground turmeric
- ½ teaspoon freshly ground black pepper
- 1 tablespoon coconut sugar (optional)

1. Preheat the oven to 400°F.
2. Brush a shallow baking dish with 1 tablespoon of ghee.
3. Place the fish fillets in the dish and brush them with the remaining 1 tablespoon of ghee.
4. In a small bowl, combine the paprika, cumin, onion powder, salt, turmeric, pepper, and coconut sugar (if using).
5. Use 1 tablespoon of the spice rub on the fillets, making sure the surface of the fish is covered with rub. Store the remaining rub for future use.
6. Place the baking dish in the preheated oven and bake the fish for 12 to 15 minutes, or until firm and cooked through.

PER SERVING

Calories: 364| Total Fat: 20g|Total Carbohydrates: 3g|Sugar: 1g| Fiber: 1g|Protein: 42g| Sodium: 1277mg

Pecan-Crusted Trout

Prep time: 5 minutes | Cook time: 15 minutes | Serves 4

- Extra-virgin olive oil, for brushing
- 4 large boneless trout fillets
- Salt
- Freshly ground black pepper
- 1 cup pecans, finely ground, divided
- 1 tablespoon coconut oil, melted, divided
- 2 tablespoon chopped fresh thyme leaves
- Lemon wedges, for garnish

1. Preheat the oven to 375°F.
2. Brush a rimmed baking sheet with olive oil.
3. Place the trout fillets on the baking sheet skin-side down. Season with salt and pepper.
4. Gently press ¼ cup of ground pecans into the flesh of each fillet.
5. Drizzle the melted coconut oil over the nuts and then sprinkle the thyme over the fillets.
6. Give each fillet another sprinkle of salt and pepper.
7. Place the sheet in the preheated oven and bake for 15 minutes, or until the fish is cooked through.

PER SERVING

Calories: 672| Total Fat: 59g|Total Carbohydrates: 13g|Sugar: 3g| Fiber: 9g|Protein: 30g| Sodium: 110mg

Sole with Vegetables in Foil Packets

Prep time: 5 minutes | Cook time: 15 minutes | Serves 4

- 4 (5-ounce) sole fillets
- Salt
- Freshly ground black pepper
- 1 zucchini, sliced thin, divided
- 1 carrot, sliced thin, divided
- 2 shallots, sliced thin, divided
- 2 tablespoons snipped fresh chives, divided
- 4 teaspoons extra-virgin olive oil, divided
- ½ cup vegetable broth, or water, divided
- Lemon wedges, for garnish

1. Preheat the oven to 425°F.
2. Tear off four 12-by-20-inch pieces of aluminum foil.
3. Place 1 fillet on one half of a foil piece. Season with salt and pepper.
4. Top the fillet with one-quarter each of the zucchini, carrot, and shallots. Sprinkle with 1½ teaspoons of chives.
5. Drizzle 1 teaspoon of olive oil and 2 tablespoons of vegetable broth over the vegetables and fish.
6. Fold the other half of the foil over the fish and vegetables, sealing the edges so the ingredients are completely encased in the packet and the contents won't leak. Place the packet on a large baking sheet.
7. Repeat steps 3 through 6 with the remaining ingredients.
8. Place the sheet in the preheated oven and bake the packets for 15 minutes, or until the fish is cooked through and the vegetables are tender.
9. Carefully peel back the foil (the escaping steam will be hot) and transfer the contents—the liquid, too—to a plate. Serve garnished with the lemon wedges.

PER SERVING

Calories: 224| Total Fat: 7g|Total Carbohydrates: 4g|Sugar: 2g| Fiber: 1g|Protein: 35g| Sodium: 205mg

Fish Sticks With Avocado Dipping Sauce

Prep time: 15 minutes | Cook time: 10 minutes | Serves 4

- For The Avocado Dipping Sauce
- 2 avocados
- ¼ cup freshly squeezed lime juice
- 2 tablespoons fresh cilantro leaves
- 2 tablespoons extra-virgin olive oil
- 1 teaspoon salt
- 1 teaspoon garlic powder
- Dash ground cumin
- Freshly ground black pepper
- For The Fish Sticks
- 1½ cups almond flour
- 1 teaspoon salt
- ½ teaspoon paprika
- ¼ teaspoon freshly ground black pepper
- 3 eggs
- ¼ cup coconut oil
- 1 pound cod fillets, cut into 4-inch-long, 1-inch-thick strips
- Juice of 1 lemon

To Make The Avocado Dipping Sauce

TO MAKE THE FISH STICKS

1. In a small shallow bowl, mix the almond flour, salt, paprika, and pepper. Whisk the eggs in another small shallow bowl.
2. Dip the fish sticks into the egg, and then into the almond flour mixture until fully coated.
3. In a large skillet over medium-high heat, heat the coconut oil.
4. One at time, place the fish sticks in the skillet. Cook for about 2 minutes per side, until lightly browned. Transfer to 2 plates.
5. To serve, sprinkle with the lemon juice and serve alongside the avocado dipping sauce.

PER SERVING

Calories: 583|Total Fat: 50g|Saturated Fat: 17g|Cholesterol: 200mg|Carbohydrates: 14g|Fiber: 8g|Protein: 25g

Sea Bass Baked with Tomatoes, Olives, and Capers

Prep time: 5 minutes | Cook time: 15 minutes | Serves 4

- 2 tablespoons extra-virgin olive oil
- 4 (5-ounce) sea bass fillets
- 1 small onion, diced
- ½ cup vegetable or chicken broth
- 1 cup canned diced tomatoes
- ½ cup pitted and chopped Kalamata olives
- 2 tablespoons capers, drained
- 2 cups packed spinach
- 1 teaspoon salt
- ¼ teaspoon freshly ground black pepper

1. Preheat the oven to 375°F.
2. In a baking dish, add the olive oil. Place the fish fillets in the dish, turning to coat both sides with the oil.
3. Top the fish with the onion, vegetable broth, tomatoes, olives, capers, spinach, salt, and pepper.
4. Cover the baking dish with aluminum foil and place it in the preheated oven. Bake for 15 minutes, or until the fish is cooked through.

PER SERVING

Calories: 273| Total Fat: 12g|Total Carbohydrates: 5g|Sugar: 2g| Fiber: 2g|Protein: 35g| Sodium: 1038mg

Smoked Trout Fried Rice
Prep time: 5 minutes | Cook time: 15 minutes | Serves 4

- 2 tablespoons toasted sesame oil
- 4 scallions, thinly sliced
- 1 teaspoon minced fresh ginger root
- 1 garlic clove, minced
- ⅛ teaspoon red pepper flakes
- 2 cups baby spinach
- ½ cup chicken or vegetable broth
- 4 cups cooked brown rice
- 1 teaspoon low-sodium soy sauce (optional)
- 8 ounces smoked trout, flaked
- ¼ cup toasted slivered almonds (optional)

1. Heat the sesame oil in a large skillet over high heat.
2. Add the scallions, ginger root, garlic, red pepper flakes, spinach, and broth. Sauté until the spinach has wilted, about 2 minutes.
3. Add the rice and stir to combine. Stir in the soy sauce (if using) and the trout.
4. Garnish with the almonds (if using) and serve.

PER SERVING

Calories: 430| Total Fat: 15g| Total Carbohydrates: 49g| Sugar: 2g| Fiber: 5g| Protein: 26g| Sodium: 2670mg

Open-Face Avocado Tuna Melts
Prep time: 15 minutes | Cook time: 10 minutes | Serves 4

- 4 slices sourdough bread
- 2 (5-ounce) cans wild-caught albacore tuna
- ¼ cup Paleo mayonnaise
- 2 tablespoons minced shallot
- 1 teaspoon freshly squeezed lemon juice
- Dash garlic powder
- Dash paprika
- 1 large avocado, cut in 8 slices
- 1 large tomato, cut in 8 slices
- ¼ cup shredded raw Parmesan cheese, divided

1. Preheat the broiler.
2. Line a baking sheet with aluminum foil.
3. Arrange the slices of bread in the prepared pan.
4. In a medium bowl, mix the tuna, mayonnaise, shallot, lemon juice, garlic powder, and paprika. Spread one-fourth of the tuna mixture on each slice of bread.
5. Top each with 2 of the avocado slices and 2 of the tomato slices.
6. Sprinkle each with 1 tablespoon of Parmesan cheese.
7. Broil for 3 to 4 minutes, watching carefully so they don't burn. Serve hot.

PER SERVING

Calories: 471|Total Fat: 27g|Saturated Fat: 4g|Cholesterol: 40mg|Carbohydrates: 31g|Fiber: 4g|Protein: 27g

Spiced Trout And Spinach
Prep time: 15 minutes | Cook time: 15 minutes | Serves 4

- Extra-virgin olive oil, for brushing
- ½ red onion, thinly sliced
- 1 (10-ounce) package frozen spinach, thawed
- 4 boneless trout fillets
- 1 teaspoon salt
- ¼ teaspoon chipotle powder
- ¼ teaspoon garlic powder
- 2 tablespoons fresh lemon juice

1. Preheat the oven to 375°F. Brush a 9-by-13-inch baking pan with olive oil.
2. Scatter the red onion and spinach in the pan.
3. Lay the trout fillets over the spinach.
4. Sprinkle the salt, chipotle powder, and garlic powder over the fish.
5. Cover with aluminum foil and bake until the trout is firm, about 15 minutes.
6. Drizzle with the lemon juice and serve.

PER SERVING

Calories: 160| Total Fat: 7g| Total Carbohydrates: 5g| Sugar: 1g| Fiber: 2g| Protein: 19g| Sodium: 670mg

Mediterranean Baked Salmon
Prep time: 5 minutes | Cook time: 25 minutes | Serves 4

- 4 (4-ounce) salmon fillets
- 3 tablespoons Pistachio Pesto
- ¼ cup chopped sun-dried tomatoes
- ¼ cup pitted, diced olives
- 2 tablespoons minced red onion
- 2 garlic cloves, minced
- Dash salt
- Fresh ground black pepper
- 1 tablespoon minced fresh basil

1. Preheat the oven to 400°F.
2. Line a baking sheet with aluminum foil.
3. Put the salmon fillets in the prepared pan, skin-side down.
4. Spread a thin layer of the pistachio pesto over the top of each fillet.
5. In a small bowl, mix the sun-dried tomatoes, olives, red onion, garlic, and salt, and season with pepper. Spread one-fourth of the tomato mixture over the pesto on each fillet.
6. Bake for 20 minutes. Remove from the oven and let rest for 5 minutes.
7. Sprinkle with the basil and serve immediately.

PER SERVING

Calories: 301|Total Fat: 17g|Saturated Fat: 2g|Cholesterol: 80mg|Carbohydrates: 6g|Fiber: 1g|Protein: 31g

Grilled Salmon Packets With Asparagus

Prep time: 15 minutes | Cook time: 20 minutes | Serves 4

- 4 (4-ounce) skinless salmon fillets
- 16 asparagus spears, tough ends trimmed
- 4 tablespoons avocado oil, divided
- 1 teaspoon garlic powder, divided
- ½ teaspoon salt, divided
- Freshly ground black pepper
- 1 lemon, thinly sliced

1. Preheat the oven to 400°F.
2. Cut 4 (12-inch) squares of parchment paper or foil and put on a work surface.
3. Place 1 salmon fillet in the center of each square and 4 asparagus spears next to each fillet. Brush the fish and asparagus with 1 tablespoon of avocado oil.
4. Sprinkle each fillet with ¼ teaspoon garlic powder and ⅛ teaspoon salt, and season with pepper.
5. Place the lemon slices on top of the fillets. Close and seal the parchment around each fillet so it forms a sealed packet.
6. Place the parchment packets on a baking sheet. Bake for 20 minutes.
7. Place a sealed parchment packet on each of 4 plates and serve hot.

PER SERVING

Calories: 339 | Total Fat: 23g | Saturated Fat: 3g | Cholesterol: 80mg | Carbohydrates: 1g | Fiber: 1g | Protein: 30g

Dill Salmon With Cucumber-Radish Salad

Prep time: 15 minutes | Cook time: 20 minutes | Serves 4

- 1 tablespoon extra-virgin olive oil, plus more for brushing
- 4 (3- to 4-ounce) boneless salmon fillets
- 2 or 3 dill sprigs, plus 2 teaspoons minced dill fronds
- 1 shallot, sliced
- ½ cup dry white wine
- 2 teaspoons salt, divided
- ¼ teaspoon freshly ground black pepper
- 2 cups sliced escarole
- 8 radishes, quartered
- 1 English cucumber, seeded and chopped
- 1 tablespoon fresh lemon juice, plus extra sliced lemons for garnish

1. Preheat the oven to 375°F. Brush a 9-inch square baking pan with olive oil.
2. Place the salmon fillets, skin-side down, in the pan. Scatter the dill sprigs and shallot over the fish, then add the wine, 1 teaspoon of salt, and the pepper.
3. Cover with aluminum foil and bake until the fish is firm, 20 to 25 minutes.
4. Transfer the salmon fillets to a plate and let them cool completely. Discard the remaining contents of the pan.
5. In a medium bowl, combine the escarole, radishes, cucumber, and minced dill. Add the lemon juice, 1 tablespoon of olive oil, and the remaining 1 teaspoon of salt. Toss well.
6. Mound the salad on four plates, top with the salmon, and garnish with the lemon slices. Serve.

PER SERVING

Calories: 361 | Total Fat: 22.9g | Total Carbohydrates: 5.4g | Sugar: 2g | Fiber: 0.7g | Protein: 27.5g | Sodium: 3,177mg

Miso Baked Salmon

Prep time: 5 minutes | Cook time: 15 minutes | Serves 4

- ¼ cup white miso
- ¼ cup apple cider
- 1 tablespoon unseasoned white rice vinegar
- 1 tablespoon toasted sesame oil
- ⅛ teaspoon ground ginger
- 4 (3- to 4-ounce) boneless salmon fillets
- 1 scallion, sliced
- ⅛ teaspoon red pepper flakes

1. Preheat the oven to 375°F.
2. In a small bowl whisk together the miso, cider, rice vinegar, sesame oil, and ginger. If the mixture is too thick, thin with a small amount of water.
3. Place the salmon fillets, skin-side down, in a 9-inch square baking pan. Pour the miso sauce over the salmon to coat evenly.
4. Bake until the salmon is firm, 15 to 20 minutes.
5. Top with the scallions and red pepper flakes and serve.

PER SERVING

Calories: 250 | Total Fat: 15g | Total Carbohydrates: 8g | Sugar: 4g | Fiber: 1g | Protein: 21g | Sodium: 820mg

Quinoa Salmon Bowl

Prep time: 15 minutes | Cook time: 15 minutes | Serves 4

- 4 cups cooked quinoa
- 1 pound cooked salmon, flaked
- 3 cups arugula
- 6 radishes, thinly sliced
- 1 zucchini, sliced into half moons
- 3 scallions, minced
- ½ cup almond oil
- 1 tablespoon apple cider vinegar
- 1 teaspoon Sriracha or other hot sauce (or more if you like it spicy)
- 1 teaspoon salt
- ½ cup toasted slivered almonds (optional)

1. Combine the quinoa, salmon, arugula, radishes, zucchini, and scallions in a large bowl.
2. Add the almond oil, vinegar, Sriracha, and salt and mix well.
3. Divide the mixture among four serving bowls, garnish with the toasted almonds (if using), and serve.

PER SERVING
Calories: 790| Total Fat: 52g| Total Carbohydrates: 45g| Sugar: 4g| Fiber: 8g| Protein: 37g| Sodium: 680mg

Salmon with Basil Gremolata

Prep time: 5 minutes | Cook time: 25 minutes | Serves 4

- 4 (5-ounce) skin-on salmon fillets
- 1 tablespoon plus
- 2 teaspoons extra-virgin olive oil, divided
- ¼ cup freshly squeezed lemon juice
- 1 teaspoon salt, plus additional for seasoning
- ¼ teaspoon freshly ground black pepper, plus additional for seasoning
- 1 bunch basil
- 1 garlic clove
- 1 tablespoon lemon zest
- 1 (8-ounce) bag mixed greens
- 1 small cucumber, halved lengthwise and sliced thin
- 1 cup sprouts (radish, onion, or sunflower)

1. Preheat the oven to 375°F.
2. In a shallow baking dish, place the salmon fillets and brush them with 2 teaspoons of olive oil.
3. Add the lemon juice. Season with 1 teaspoon of salt and ¼ teaspoon of pepper.
4. Place the dish in the preheated oven and bake the fillets for about 20 minutes, or until firm and cooked through.
5. In a food processor, combine the basil, garlic, and lemon zest. Process until coarsely chopped.
6. Arrange the greens, cucumber, and sprouts on a serving platter. Drizzle the greens with the remaining 2 tablespoons of olive oil and season with salt and pepper. Place the salmon fillets on top of the greens and spoon the gremolata over the salmon.

PER SERVING
Calories: 274| Total Fat: 12g|Total Carbohydrates: 11g|Sugar: 5g| Fiber: 5g|Protein: 32g| Sodium: 908mg

Salmon & Asparagus Skewers

Prep time: 15 minutes | Cook time: 10 minutes|Makes 8 skewers

- 2 tablespoons ghee, melted
- 1 teaspoon Dijon mustard
- 1 teaspoon garlic powder
- ½ teaspoon salt
- ¼ teaspoon red pepper flakes
- 1½ pounds boned skinless salmon, cut into 2-inch chunks
- 2 lemons, thinly sliced
- 1 bunch asparagus spears, tough ends trimmed, cut into 2-inch pieces

1. Preheat the broiler.
2. Line a baking sheet with aluminum foil.
3. In a small saucepan over medium heat, heat the ghee.
4. Stir in the mustard, garlic powder, salt, and red pepper flakes.
5. On each skewer, thread 1 chunk of salmon, 1 lemon slice folded in half, and 2 pieces of asparagus. Repeat with the remaining skewers until all ingredients are used. Place the skewers on the prepared pan and brush each with the ghee-seasoning mixture.
6. Broil for 4 minutes. Turn the skewers and broil on the other side for about 4 minutes.

PER SERVING
Calories: 250|Total Fat: 9g|Saturated Fat: 5g|Cholesterol: 68mg|Carbohydrates: 4g|Fiber: 2g|Protein: 38g

Coconut-Crusted Cod With Mango-Pineapple Salsa

Prep time: 5 minutes | Cook time: 20 minutes| Serves 4

- For The Salsa
- 1 cup diced mango
- 1 cup diced pineapple
- ½ large avocado, diced
- Juice of 1 lime
- Dash salt
- Dash chili powder
- For The Cod
- 1 egg
- 1 cup unsweetened dried coconut
- 2 tablespoons avocado oil
- 4 (4-ounce) cod fillets
- 1 teaspoon salt
- ½ teaspoon garlic powder
- ¼ teaspoon cayenne pepper

TO MAKE THE SALSA

To Make The Cod
1. In a small shallow bowl, beat the egg. Put the coconut in another small shallow bowl.
2. Dip each cod fillet into the egg, then into the coconut until well coated, and place on a plate.
3. Sprinkle each fillet with the salt, garlic powder, and cayenne pepper.
4. In a large skillet over medium-high heat, heat the avocado oil.
5. Cook each fillet one at a time in the hot skillet for 4 to 5 minutes. Flip and cook on the other side for 1 to 2 minutes until the flesh begins to flake. Transfer to a plate.
6. Top each fillet with salsa and serve.

PER SERVING

Calories: 369|Total Fat: 27g|Saturated Fat: 14g|Cholesterol: 107mg|Carbohydrates: 18g|Fiber: 5g|Protein: 18g

Curried Poached Halibut

Prep time: 5 minutes | Cook time: 24 minutes| Serves 4

- 1 tablespoon avocado oil
- ½ cup diced white onion
- 2 garlic cloves, minced
- 1 tablespoon red curry paste
- 1½ cups chicken broth
- 1 (14-ounce) can coconut milk
- ½ teaspoon coconut sugar
- 1 teaspoon salt
- ½ teaspoon freshly ground black pepper
- 4 (4-ounce) halibut fillets

1. In a large skillet over medium heat, heat the avocado oil.
2. Add the onion and garlic, and sauté for 2 to 3 minutes until the onions are translucent.
3. Stir in the curry paste until incorporated.
4. Add the broth, coconut milk, coconut sugar, salt, and pepper and stir to combine. Reduce the heat to medium-low and gently simmer for 10 minutes.
5. Pat the halibut dry with a paper towel. Place each fillet into the curried broth. Cover and poach for 10 minutes. Check the fish for doneness|if it flakes, it should be done. To speed the cooking time, occasionally spoon some broth over the halibut as it cooks.
6. Serve the fillets in four bowls with the curried broth spooned on top.

PER SERVING

Calories: 358|Total Fat: 22g|Saturated Fat: 17g|Cholesterol: 68mg|Carbohydrates: 10g|Fiber: 1g|Protein: 28g

Chapter 12
Poultry & Meat Dishes

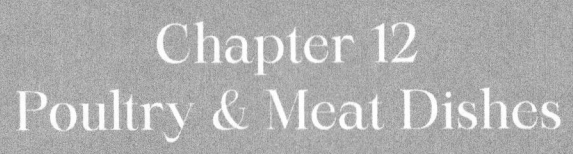

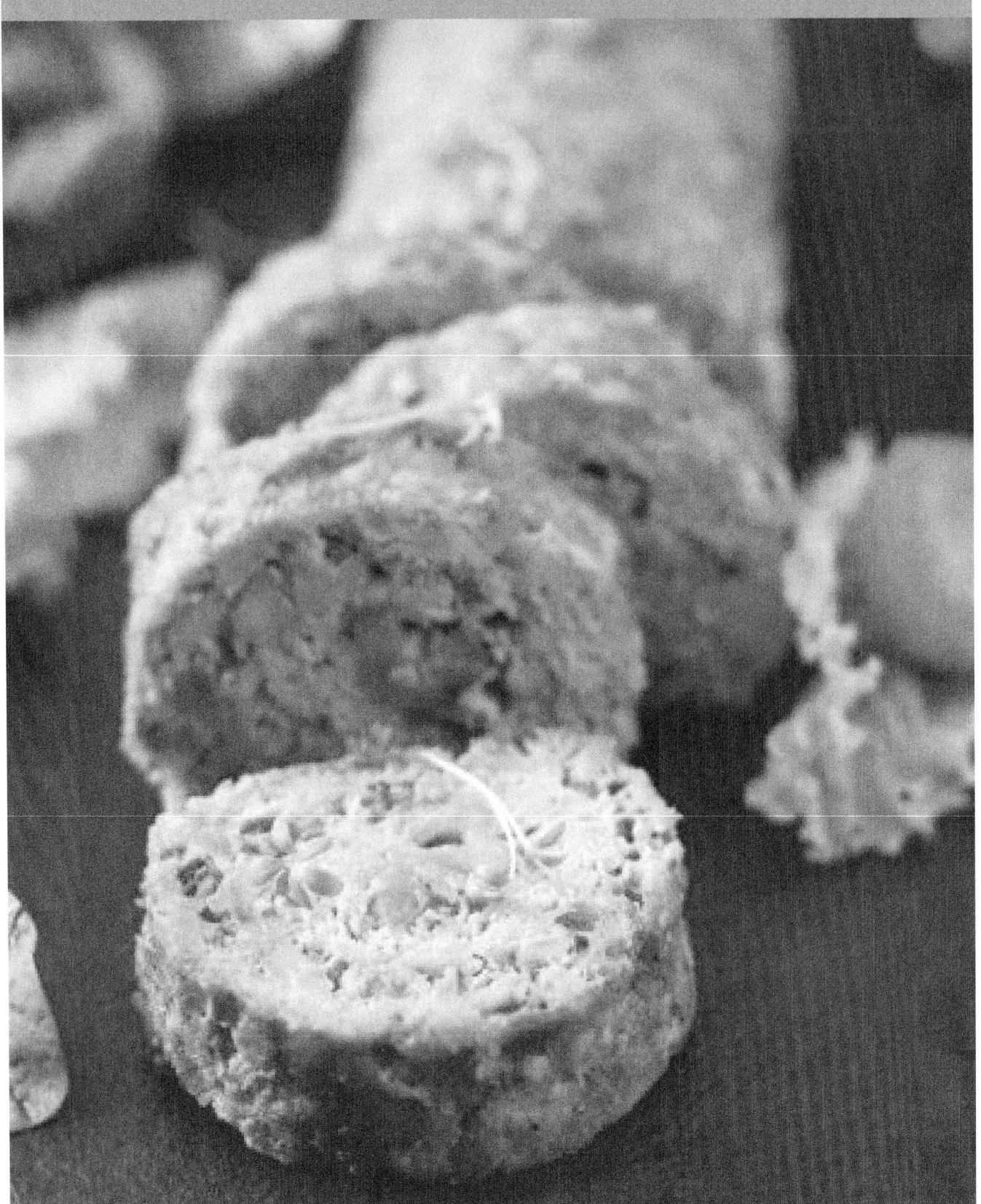

Turkey Larb Lettuce Wraps

Prep time: 10 minutes | Cooking time: 20 minutes | Serves 4

- 1 pound ground turkey
- 1 small red onion, diced
- 2 garlic cloves, minced
- 4 scallions, sliced
- 2 tablespoons freshly squeezed lime juice
- 2 tablespoons fish sauce
- 2 tablespoons minced fresh cilantro
- 1 tablespoon minced fresh mint (optional)
- 1 tablespoon coconut sugar
- ¼ teaspoon red pepper flakes
- 8 small romaine lettuce leaves

1. In a large skillet over medium-high heat, cook the turkey for 10 minutes, stirring and breaking up the meat.
2. Add the onion and garlic, and cook for about 10 minutes, stirring, until the onions soften and the meat is cooked.
3. Remove from the heat. Stir in the scallions, lime juice, fish sauce, cilantro, mint (if using), coconut sugar, and red pepper flakes until well incorporated.
4. Fill each romaine leaf with the meat mixture.
5. Serve warm or cold.

PER SERVING

Calories 143 | Total Fat 2g | Saturated Fat 1g | Cholesterol 70mg | Carbohydrates 9g | Fiber 1g | Protein 24g

Indonesian Chicken Satay

Prep time: 15 minutes plus 1 hour to marinate | Cook time: 10 minutes | Serves 4

- For The Sauce
- ½ cup almond butter
- ¼ cup water
- 2 tablespoons coconut aminos
- 1 tablespoon grated fresh ginger
- 1 tablespoon freshly squeezed lime juice
- 1 garlic clove
- 1 teaspoon raw honey
- For The Satay
- Juice of 2 limes (2 to 4 tablespoons)
- 2 tablespoons olive oil
- 2 tablespoons raw honey
- 1 tablespoon finely chopped fresh cilantro
- 1 tablespoon bottled minced garlic
- 1½ pounds boneless skinless chicken breast, cut into strips

TO MAKE THE SAUCE

In a blender, combine the almond butter, water, coconut aminos, ginger, lime juice, garlic, and honey. Pulse until smooth. Set it aside.

TO MAKE THE SATAY

1. In a large bowl, whisk the lime juice, olive oil, honey, cilantro, and garlic until well mixed.
2. Add the chicken strips and toss to coat. Cover the bowl with plastic wrap and refrigerate for 1 hour to marinate.
3. Preheat the broiler.
4. Place a rack in the upper quarter of the oven.
5. Thread each chicken strip onto a wooden skewer, and lay them on a rimmed baking sheet.
6. Broil the chicken for about 4 minutes per side until cooked through and golden, turning once.
7. Serve with the sauce.

PER SERVING

Calories: 181 | Total fat: 11g | Saturated fat: 2g | Carbohydrates: 12g | Fiber: 0g | Protein: 10g

Brown Rice Congee

Prep time: 15 minutes | Cook time: 10 minutes | Serves 6

- 2½ cups brown rice, rinsed well
- 7 to 8 cups Basic Chicken Broth, plus additional as needed
- 1-inch piece fresh ginger, grated
- 1 teaspoon salt
- 3 cups lightly packed spinach leaves
- 2 tablespoons toasted sesame oil (optional)

1. In a large pot set over high heat, combine the rice, broth, ginger, and salt. Bring to a boil, then reduce the heat to low. Cover and cook for 1½ to 2 hours, stirring occasionally. If the congee becomes too thick, add additional broth.
2. When the congee is cooked, stir in the spinach and let it wilt for about 5 minutes.
3. Drizzle with sesame oil (if using) and serve.

PER SERVING

Calories: 384 | Total Fat: 9g | Total Carbohydrates: 63g | Sugar: 1g | Fiber: 13g | Protein: 13g | Sodium: 1033mg

Turkey Chili

Prep time: 15 minutes | Cook time: 65 minutes | Serves 6

- 2 onions, finely diced
- 8 garlic cloves, minced
- 2 tablespoons water
- 1½ pounds ground turkey
- 6 cups crushed or diced tomatoes
- 2 tablespoons chili powder, plus additional as needed
- 1 teaspoon salt, plus additional as needed

1. In a large pot set over medium heat, sauté the onions and garlic with the water for about 5 minutes, or until soft.
2. Add the ground turkey, breaking it up with a spoon, and cook for 5 minutes more.
3. Stir in the tomatoes, chili powder, and salt. Bring to a boil. Reduce the heat to low. Cover and simmer for 45 minutes, stirring occasionally. If the chili gets too dry, add more water.
4. Taste and adjust the seasoning, if necessary.

PER SERVING

Calories: 350| Total Fat: 13g| Total Carbohydrates: 26g| Sugar: 16g| Fiber: 10g| Protein: 38g| Sodium: 1016mg

Glazed Chicken With Broccoli

Prep time: 15 minutes | Cook time: 40 minutes | Serves 6

- ¼ cup coconut oil, divided
- 1 pound chicken breasts, cut into chunks
- ¼ cup raw honey
- 3 broccoli heads, chopped
- 1 teaspoon salt
- 2 tablespoons sesame seeds

1. Preheat the oven to 350°F.
2. In a large ovenproof dish or pot set over medium heat, heat 2 tablespoons of coconut oil.
3. Add the chicken. Sauté for 10 minutes.
4. Stir in the honey until well combined. Turn off the heat.
5. Add the broccoli to the pot.
6. Sprinkle with the salt.
7. Cover the pot and place it into the preheated oven. Bake for 20 minutes. Remove the lid and cook for 5 minutes more.
8. Sprinkle with the sesame seeds and serve.

PER SERVING

Calories: 470| Total Fat: 25g| Total Carbohydrates: 28g| Sugar: 20g| Fiber: 4g| Protein: 38g| Sodium: 725mg

Apple-Turkey Burgers

Prep time: 15 minutes | Cook time: 30 minutes | Serves 6

- 1 red onion, finely chopped
- 1 apple, washed and grated
- 1 pound ground turkey
- ¼ cup chickpea flour, plus additional as needed
- ½ teaspoon salt

1. Preheat the oven to 350°F.
2. Line a baking sheet with parchment paper.
3. In a large bowl, combine the onion and apple.
4. Add the ground turkey, chickpea flour, and salt. Mix well. If your mixture seems too wet, add another 1 or 2 tablespoons of chickpea flour.
5. Using a ⅓-cup measure, scoop the turkey mixture onto the prepared sheet. Flatten the patties with the bottom of the measure so they are ¾ to 1 inch thick.
6. Place the sheet in the preheated oven and bake for 30 minutes, or until the burgers are cooked through, are opaque in the middle, and the internal temperature reaches 165°F.

PER SERVING

Calories: 301| Total Fat: 13g| Total Carbohydrates: 16g| Sugar: 7g| Fiber: 4g| Protein: 34g| Sodium: 417mg

Turkey-Thyme Meatballs

Prep time: 15 minutes | Cook time: 20 minutes | Serves 4

- Make Ahead
- 1½ pounds lean ground turkey
- ½ sweet onion, chopped, or about ½ cup precut packaged onion
- ¼ cup almond flour
- 1 tablespoon chopped fresh thyme
- 2 teaspoons bottled minced garlic
- 1 egg
- ¼ teaspoon ground nutmeg
- Pinch sea salt

1. Preheat the oven to 350°F.
2. Line a rimmed baking sheet with aluminum foil and set it aside.
3. In a large bowl, combine the turkey, onion, almond flour, thyme, garlic, egg, nutmeg, and sea salt until well mixed. Roll the turkey mixture into 1½-inch meatballs. Arrange the meatballs on the prepared baking sheet.
4. Bake for about 15 minutes, or until browned and cooked through.

PER SERVING

Calories: 303|Total fat: 16g|Saturated fat: 4g|Carbohydrates: 4g|Fiber: 1g|Protein: 36g

Slow-Cooker Chicken Alfredo

Prep time: 15 minutes | Cook time: 4-8 hours | Serves 6

- 1 large cauliflower head, broken or cut into florets
- Heaping ½ cup cashews, soaked in water for at least 4 hours
- 1 teaspoon salt
- ¼ cup water, reserved from cooking the cauliflower
- 6 (2- to 3-ounce) bone-in skinless chicken thighs
- 4 cups spinach

TO MAKE THE SAUCE

1. Fill a large pot with 2 inches of water and insert a steamer basket. Bring to a boil over high heat.
2. In a colander, drain and rinse the cashews.
3. In a blender, combine the cooked cauliflower, cashews, salt, and ¼ cup of the cauliflower cooking liquid. Blend until smooth and creamy.

TO MAKE THE CHICKEN

4. Place the chicken thighs in a slow cooker.
5. Pour the sauce over the chicken.
6. Cook on high for 3 to 4 hours, or on low for 7 to 8 hours.
7. Transfer the chicken to a work surface. Remove and discard the bones and gristle. Shred the chicken meat.
8. Return the chicken meat to the cooker.
9. Stir in the spinach. Cook for about 5 minutes, or until the spinach wilts.

PER SERVING

Calories: 286| Total Fat: 18g| Total Carbohydrates: 12g| Sugar: 4g| Fiber: 4g| Protein: 27g| Sodium: 511mg

Lamb-Stuffed Peppers

Prep time: 15 minutes | Cook time: 65 minutes | Serves 8

- 1 onion, finely diced
- 2 tablespoons water, plus additional for cooking
- 1½ pounds ground lamb
- 1 cup grated zucchini (about 1 zucchini)
- ¼ cup fresh basil, minced
- 1 teaspoon salt
- 6 bell peppers, any color, seeded, ribbed, tops removed and reserved

1. Preheat the oven to 350°F.
2. In a large pan set over medium heat, sauté the onion in the water for about 5 minutes, or until soft.
3. Add the ground lamb and zucchini. Cook for 10 minutes, breaking up the meat with a spoon.
4. Stir in the basil and salt. Remove from the heat.
5. Fill a casserole dish with 1½ inches of water.
6. Stuff each pepper with an equal amount of the lamb mixture and place them into the dish. Cap each pepper with its reserved top.
7. Place the dish in the preheated oven and bake for 45 to 50 minutes.

PER SERVING

Calories: 258| Total Fat: 9g| Total Carbohydrates: 10g| Sugar: 6g| Fiber: 3g| Protein: 34g| Sodium: 481mg

Baked Turkey Meatballs With Zucchini Noodles

Prep time: 15 minutes | Cook time: 30 minutes | Serves 6

- 4 zucchini
- ½ cup extra-virgin olive oil
- ½ cup fresh basil
- 3 tablespoons chickpea flour
- 1 teaspoon salt

1. Using a spiral slicer, spiralize the zucchini into noodles. You can also use a vegetable peeler to slice them into thin strips. Transfer to a large serving bowl.
2. In a blender, blend together the olive oil and basil. Drizzle over the noodles.

TO MAKE THE MEATBALLS

3. Preheat the oven to 350°F.
4. Line a baking sheet with parchment paper.
5. In a medium bowl, mix together the ground turkey, chickpea flour, and salt.
6. Using 1 tablespoon for each, roll the mixture into meatballs and place them on the prepared sheet.
7. Place the sheet in the preheated oven and bake for 20 to 25 minutes, or until lightly browned and cooked through.
8. Combine the meatballs with the zucchini noodles and serve.

PER SERVING

Calories: 444| Total Fat: 34g| Total Carbohydrates: 12g| Sugar: 4g| Fiber: 4g| Protein: 27g| Sodium: 689mg

Coconut Chicken Curry

Prep time: 15 minutes | Cook time: 40 minutes | Serves 6

- 3 cups coconut milk
- 2 cups water
- 1 to 2 tablespoons curry powder
- 2 pounds boneless skinless chicken thighs, cut into cubes
- 1 teaspoon salt
- 3 bunches Swiss chard, washed, stemmed, and roughly chopped

1. In a large pot, combine the coconut milk, water, curry powder, chicken, and salt. Bring to a boil over high heat. Reduce the heat to low. Cover and simmer for 30 minutes.
2. Add the Swiss chard to the pot. Cook for 5 minutes, or until the chard wilts.

PER SERVING

Calories: 581| Total Fat: 40g| Total Carbohydrates: 10g| Sugar: 5g| Fiber: 4g| Protein: 48g| Sodium: 652mg

Chicken Sliders

Prep time: 15 minutes | Cook time: 30 minutes| Serves 6

- ¼ cup quinoa flour, brown rice flour, or chickpea flour
- 1 pound ground chicken
- 4 scallions, finely sliced
- ¾ teaspoon salt
- 2 to 4 tablespoons coconut oil, divided

1. Cover a large plate with parchment paper.
2. In a medium bowl, mix together the quinoa flour and chicken. In a medium bowl, mix together the quinoa flour and the chicken. Fold in the scallions and add the salt.
3. With wet hands, take about 2 tablespoons of the chicken mixture and roll into a ball. Flatten into a patty and place it on the prepared plate. Repeat with the remaining mixture.
4. In a large sauté pan set over medium heat, heat 2 tablespoons of coconut oil.
5. Add the patties, working in batches, and cook for 8 to10 minutes per side. Add more oil to the pan, if needed, for additional batches. Fully cooked patties should register at least 165°F on a meat thermometer.
6. Serve hot.

PER SERVING

Calories: 365| Total Fat: 23g| Total Carbohydrates: 3g| Sugar: 0g| Fiber: 0g| Protein: 37g| Sodium: 538mg

Sesame Chicken Stir-Fry

Prep time: 15 minutes | Cook time: 30 minutes| Serves 8

- ¾ cup warm water
- ½ cup tahini
- ¼ cup plus 2 tablespoons toasted sesame oil, divided
- 2 garlic cloves, minced
- ½ teaspoon salt
- 1 pound boneless skinless chicken breasts, cut into ½-inch cubes
- 6 cups lightly packed kale, thoroughly washed and chopped

1. In a medium bowl, whisk together the warm water, tahini, ¼ cup of sesame oil, garlic, and salt.
2. In a large pan set over medium heat, heat the remaining 2 tablespoons of sesame oil.
3. Add the chicken and cook for 8 to 10 minutes, stirring.
4. Stir in the tahini-sesame sauce, mixing well to coat the chicken. Cook for 6 to 8 minutes more.
5. One handful at a time, add the kale. When the first handful wilts, add the next. Continue until all the kale has been added. Serve hot.

PER SERVING

Calories: 417| Total Fat: 30g| Total Carbohydrates: 12g| Sugar: 0g| Fiber: 3g| Protein: 27g| Sodium: 311mg

Lamb Souvlaki

Prep time: 15 minutes plus 1 hour marinating | Cook time: 20 minutes|Makes 8 skewers

- 2 tablespoons olive oil
- 2 tablespoons apple cider vinegar
- 1 tablespoon dried oregano
- 2 teaspoons bottled minced garlic
- ½ teaspoon sea salt
- 1 pound lamb shoulder, cut into 1-inch cubes

1. In a large bowl, stir together the olive oil, cider vinegar, oregano, garlic, and sea salt until well mixed.
2. Stir in the lamb. Cover the bowl and refrigerate it for 1 hour to marinate.
3. Preheat the broiler.
4. Place one of the racks in the upper third of the oven.
5. Using 8 wooden skewers, thread 4 or 5 pieces of lamb on each and arrange them on a baking sheet.
6. Broil, turning, for about 15 minutes total until the meat is browned evenly on all sides.

PER SERVING

Calories: 278|Total fat: 15g|Saturated fat: 4g|Carbohydrates: 1g|Fiber: 1g|Protein: 32g

Coconut Braised Chicken

Prep time: 15 minutes | Cook time: 35 minutes| Serves 4

- 1½ cups canned lite coconut milk
- 2 tablespoons grated fresh ginger
- Juice of 1 lime (1 or 2 tablespoons)
- Zest of 1 lime (optional)
- 1 tablespoon raw honey
- ½ teaspoon ground cardamom
- 1 tablespoon olive oil
- 1 pound bone-in skin-on chicken thighs
- 1 scallion, white and green parts, chopped

1. In a medium bowl, whisk the coconut milk, ginger, lime juice, lime zest (if using), honey, and cardamom. Set it aside.
2. Place a large skillet over medium-high heat and add the olive oil.
3. Add the chicken thighs and pan-sear for about 20 minutes, or until golden, turning once.
4. Pour the coconut milk mixture over the chicken, and bring the liquid to a boil. Reduce the heat to low, cover, and simmer for about 15 minutes, or until the chicken is tender and cooked through.
5. Serve garnished with the scallions.

PER SERVING

Calories: 480|Total fat: 34g|Saturated fat: 22g|Carbohydrates: 12g|Fiber: 3g|Protein: 35g

Chicken Buckwheat Florentine

Prep time: 15 minutes | Cook time: 45 minutes | Serves 6

- Make Ahead
- 1 tablespoon olive oil
- 3 (8-ounce) boneless skinless chicken breasts, diced
- 1 sweet onion, chopped, or about 1 cup precut packaged onion
- 2 cups sliced button mushrooms
- 2 teaspoons bottled minced garlic
- 1 cup uncooked buckwheat
- 1 cup Herbed Chicken Bone Broth
- 1 cup canned lite coconut milk
- ½ teaspoon ground nutmeg
- 4 cups fresh spinach
- Sea salt
- Zest of 1 lemon (optional)

1. Place a skillet over medium-high heat and add the olive oil.
2. Add the chicken. Sauté for about 15 minutes, turning once, until just cooked through. With a slotted spoon, remove the chicken to a plate and set it aside. Return the skillet to the heat.
3. Add the onion, mushrooms, and garlic to the skillet. Sauté for about 5 minutes, or until softened.
4. Pour in the buckwheat and sauté for 1 minute.
5. Stir in the chicken broth, coconut milk, and nutmeg. Bring the liquid to a boil. Reduce the heat to low and simmer, covered, for about 25 minutes, or until the buckwheat is tender.
6. Stir in the spinach and chicken, and season with sea salt.
7. Serve sprinkled with lemon zest (if using).

PER SERVING

Calories: 490 | Total fat: 22g | Saturated fat: 11g | Carbohydrates: 37g | Fiber: 6g | Protein: 40g

Bubbie's Comforting Chicken Soup

Prep time: 15 minutes | Cook time: about 2 hours | Serves 6

- 10 bone-in skinless chicken pieces, a mix of legs and thighs (about 3 pounds total)
- 8 to 10 cups water, divided
- 1 large onion, washed
- 4 carrots, peeled and chopped
- 4 celery stalks, chopped
- 1 bunch fresh parsley, stemmed and minced
- 1 teaspoon salt, plus additional as needed

1. In a large pot set over high heat, combine the chicken with 8 cups of water.
2. Add the whole onion to the pot.
3. Bring to a boil. Reduce the heat to medium-low. Cover and cook for 1 hour. If scum rises to the top, skim it off.
4. After 1 hour, remove the onion from the pot. Add the carrots, celery, parsley, and salt. Cover the pot and simmer the soup for 30 minutes more. Add some of the remaining 2 cups of water, as needed.
5. Remove the chicken from the pot. Debone and shred the meat.
6. Return the chicken meat to the pot.
7. Stir, taste, adjust the seasoning if needed, and serve.

PER SERVING

Calories: 471 | Total Fat: 36g | Total Carbohydrates: 7g | Sugar: 3g | Fiber: 2g | Protein: 31g | Sodium: 592mg

Pork Tenderloin With Savory Berry Sauce

Prep time: 15 minutes | Cook time: 20 minutes plus 10 minutes resting | Serves 4

- For The Pork
- 2 (10-ounce) pork tenderloins, trimmed and patted dry
- Sea salt
- Freshly ground black pepper
- 1 tablespoon olive oil

TO MAKE THE PORK

1. Preheat the oven to 425°F.
2. Place a medium ovenproof skillet over medium-high heat and add the olive oil.
3. Add the pork. Brown it on all sides, turning, for about 5 minutes total.
4. Place the skillet in the oven and roast the pork for about 15 minutes until just cooked through. Remove from the oven and let the pork rest for 10 minutes.
5. Slice the pork into medallions and serve with the berry sauce.

FOR THE SAUCE

- 1 tablespoon olive oil
- ¼ cup finely chopped sweet onion
- 2 tablespoons apple cider vinegar
- 1 cup fresh blueberries
- ¼ teaspoon ground nutmeg
- 1 teaspoon lemon zest (optional)

TO MAKE THE SAUCE

1. While the pork roasts, place a small saucepan over medium-high heat and add the olive oil.
2. Add the onion. Sauté for about 3 minutes, or until softened.
3. Stir in the chicken broth and cider vinegar. Bring the liquid to a boil. Reduce the heat to low and simmer for about 4 minutes, or until the sauce has reduced by half.
4. Stir in the blueberries and nutmeg. Cook for about 5 minutes, or until the berries break down. Remove the sauce from the heat and stir in the lemon zest (if using).
5. Serve with the pork medallions.

PER SERVING

Calories: 375 | Total fat: 19g | Saturated fat: 5g | Carbohydrates: 6g | Fiber: 1g | Protein: 43g

Pork Chops With Cooked Apple Salsa

Prep time: 15 minutes | Cook time: 30 minutes | Serves 4

- For The Salsa
- 1 teaspoon olive oil
- ¼ cup finely chopped sweet onion
- ½ teaspoon grated fresh ginger
- 2 apples, peeled, cored, and diced
- ½ cup dried raisins
- Pinch sea salt
- For The Pork Chops
- 4 (4-ounce) boneless center-cut pork chops, trimmed and patted dry
- 1 teaspoon garlic powder
- 1 teaspoon ground cinnamon
- Sea salt
- Freshly ground black pepper
- 1 tablespoon olive oil

TO MAKE THE SALSA

1. Place a medium skillet over medium heat and add the olive oil.
2. Add the onion and ginger. Sauté for about 2 minutes, or until softened.
3. Stir in the apples and raisins. Sauté for about 5 minutes, or until the fruit is just tender. Season the salsa with sea salt and set it aside.

TO MAKE THE PORK CHOPS

1. Sprinkle the pork chops on both sides with the garlic powder, cinnamon, sea salt, and pepper.
2. Place a large skillet over medium-high heat and add the olive oil.
3. Add the seasoned chops and panfry for 7 to 8 minutes per side until just cooked through and browned, turning once.
4. Serve the chops with the cooked apple salsa.

PER SERVING

Calories: 434|Total fat: 32g|Saturated fat: 11g|Carbohydrates: 10g|Fiber: 1g|Protein: 26g

Grainy Mustard Crusted Lamb

Prep time: 15 minutes | Cook time: 35 minutes plus 10 minutes resting | Serves 4

- ¼ cup whole-grain Dijon mustard
- 2 tablespoons chopped fresh thyme
- 1 tablespoon chopped fresh rosemary
- 2 (8-rib) frenched lamb racks, patted dry
- Sea salt
- Freshly ground black pepper
- 1 tablespoon olive oil

1. Preheat the oven to 425°F.
2. In a small bowl, stir together the mustard, thyme, and rosemary.
3. Lightly season the lamb racks with sea salt and pepper.
4. Place a large ovenproof skillet over medium-high heat and add the olive oil.
5. Add the lamb racks. Pan-sear for about 2 minutes per side, turning once. Remove the skillet from the heat.
6. Turn the racks upright in the skillet with the bones interlaced, and spread the mustard mixture over the outside surface of the lamb. Roast for about 30 minutes for medium, or until your desired doneness.
7. Remove the lamb racks from the oven and let them rest for 10 minutes. Cut the racks into chops and serve 4 per person.

PER SERVING

Calories: 469|Total fat: 21g|Saturated fat: 7g|Carbohydrates: 2g|Fiber: 1g|Protein: 65g

Moroccan Lamb Stew

Prep time: 15 minutes | Cook time: 2 hours, 15 minutes | Serves 4

- Make Ahead
- 2 tablespoons olive oil, divided
- 1 pound lamb shoulder, trimmed of visible fat and cut into 1-inch chunks
- 2 stalks celery, chopped, or about ¾ to 1 cup precut packaged celery
- 1 sweet onion, chopped, or about 1 cup precut packaged onion
- 1 tablespoon grated fresh ginger
- 2 teaspoons bottled minced garlic
- 1 teaspoon ground cinnamon
- ½ teaspoon ground turmeric
- ¼ teaspoon ground allspice
- 2 cups Beef Bone Broth
- 2 cups diced sweet potato
- 1 cup diced carrot
- 1 cup diced parsnip
- 2 cups fresh spinach
- 2 tablespoons chopped fresh parsley

1. Preheat the oven to 325°F.
2. Place a large ovenproof skillet over medium-high heat and add 1 tablespoon of olive oil.
3. Add the lamb in batches. Brown for about 8 minutes total. With a slotted spoon, remove the meat to a plate. Return the skillet to the heat.
4. To the skillet, add the remaining 1 tablespoon of olive oil, the celery, onion, ginger, and garlic. Sauté for about 3 minutes, or until softened.
5. Stir in the cinnamon, turmeric, and allspice. Sauté for 1 minute.
6. Stir in the beef broth, lamb, and any accumulated juices on the plate, the sweet potato, carrot, and parsnip. Bring the liquid to a boil. Cover the skillet and place it in the oven. Braise the stew for about 2 hours, stirring occasionally, until the lamb is very tender.
7. Remove the stew from the oven and stir in the spinach.
8. Let the stew sit for 10 minutes. Serve garnished with the parsley.

PER SERVING

Calories: 432|Total fat: 16g|Saturated fat: 4g|Carbohydrates: 35g|Fiber: 7g|Protein: 37g

Savory Beef Meatloaf

Prep time: 15 minutes | Cook time: 1 hour plus 10 minutes resting | Serves 4

- 1½ pounds extra-lean ground beef
- ½ cup almond flour
- ½ cup chopped sweet onion
- 1 egg
- 1 tablespoon chopped fresh basil
- 1 tablespoon chopped fresh parsley
- 1 teaspoon grated fresh horseradish, or prepared horseradish
- ⅛ teaspoon sea salt

1. Preheat the oven to 350°F.
2. In a large bowl, combine the ground beef, almond flour, onion, egg, basil, parsley, horseradish, and sea salt until well mixed. Press the meatloaf mixture into a 9-by-5-inch loaf pan.
3. Bake for about 1 hour until cooked through.
4. Remove the meatloaf from the oven, and let it rest for 10 minutes.

PER SERVING

Calories: 407|Total fat: 18g|Saturated fat: 5g|Carbohydrates: 4g|Fiber: 2g|Protein: 56g

Buckwheat Cabbage Rolls

Prep time: 15 minutes | Cook time: 1 hour, 5 minutes | Serves 4

- 8 large outer cabbage leaves with the hard core removed
- 1 pound lean ground beef
- ½ cup cooked buckwheat
- ½ sweet onion, chopped, or about ½ cup precut packaged onion
- 1 egg
- 2 teaspoons bottled minced garlic
- 1 teaspoon chopped fresh oregano
- Pinch sea salt
- ½ cup Beef Bone Broth

1. Preheat the oven to 350°F.
2. Fill a large saucepan with water, place it over high heat, and bring to a boil.
3. Add the cabbage leaves. Blanch for about 4 minutes, or until tender. Remove them from the water and set them aside.
4. In a large bowl, combine the ground beef, buckwheat, onion, egg, garlic, oregano, and sea salt until well mixed. Divide the mixture into 8 portions.
5. Place 1 cabbage leaf on a work surface, and place 1 meat portion in the center. Fold the sides of the leaf over the meat. Roll the leaf from the nearest unfolded edge until the meat is completely enclosed in a roll. Place the roll seam-side down in a 9-by-9-inch baking dish. Repeat with the remaining leaves and meat portions.
6. Pour the beef broth over the cabbage rolls. Cover the baking dish with aluminum foil, and bake for about 1 hour until the filling is cooked through.

PER SERVING

Calories: 380|Total fat: 8g|Saturated fat: 3g|Carbohydrates: 35g|Fiber: 5g|Protein: 41g

Chapter 13
Snacks, Appetizers, and Savory Fat Bombs

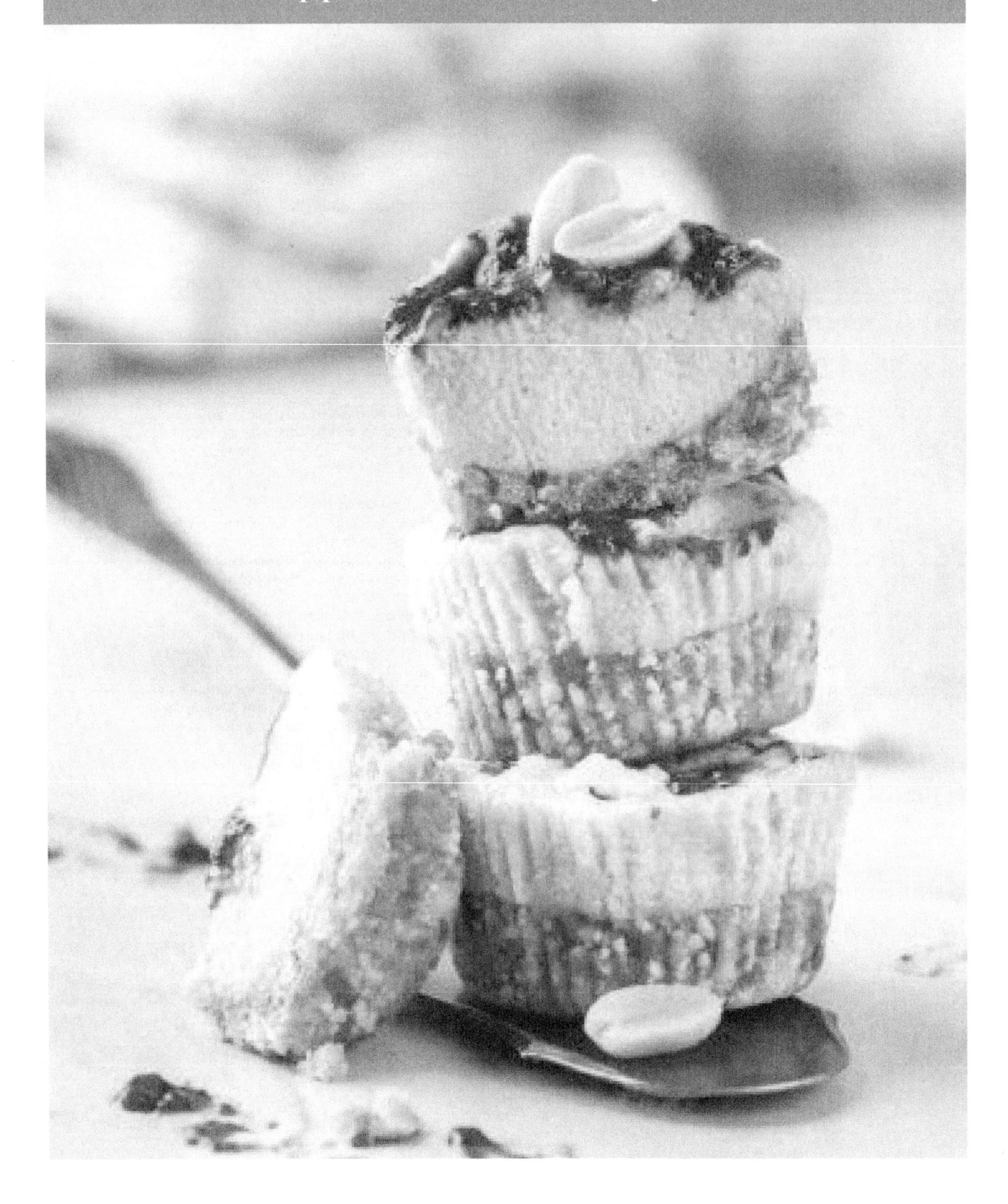

Mushroom Bites

Prep time: 5 minutes | Cook time: 12 minutes | Serves 8

- Salt and black pepper to the taste
- 1 and ¼ cups coconut flour
- 2 garlic clove, minced
- 2 tablespoons basil, minced
- ½ pound mushrooms, minced
- 1 egg, whisked

1. In a bowl, mix all the ingredients except the Cooking spray, stir well and shape medium balls out of this mix.
2. Arrange the balls in your air fryer's basket, grease them with Cooking spray and bake at 350 degrees F for 6 minutes on each side. Serve as an appetizer.

PER SERVING

Calories 151|Fat 2|Fiber 1|Carbs 3|Protein 6

Roasted Garlic Mushrooms

Prep time: 5 minutes| Cook time:25 minutes | Serves 4

- Nonstick cooking spray
- 1⅓ pounds cremini mushrooms
- 6 garlic cloves, minced
- 3 tablespoons avocado oil
- 3 tablespoons Parmesan cheese
- ½ teaspoon salt
- ¼ teaspoon freshly ground black pepper
- 3 tablespoons dried parsley

1. Preheat the oven to 400°F. Line a baking sheet with aluminum foil and spray with nonstick cooking spray.
2. In a mixing bowl, combine the mushrooms, garlic, avocado oil, Parmesan cheese, salt, and pepper. Mix well.
3. Spread the mushroom mixture on the prepared baking sheet and sprinkle with the parsley.
4. Bake for 12 minutes and stir. Return to the oven and bake for an additional 12 minutes.
5. Transfer the mushrooms to a serving dish.

PER SERVING (⅓ CUP)

Calories: 180|Fat: 13g|Protein: 8g|Total carbs: 8g|Net carbs: 7g|Fiber: 1g|Sugar: 3g|Sodium: 400mg Macros: Fat: 66%|Protein: 17%|Carbs: 17%

Smoked Almonds

Prep time: 5 minutes| Cook time:45 minutes| Serves 10

- 1 pound raw almonds
- 2 tablespoons grass-fed butter, melted
- 2 tablespoons liquid smoke
- 2 tablespoons Worcestershire sauce
- 1 tablespoon salt

1. Preheat the oven to 200°F. Line a baking dish with aluminum foil.
2. Put the almonds in a large mixing bowl and set aside.
3. In a small bowl, mix together the butter, liquid smoke, and Worcestershire sauce.
4. Pour the mixture over the almonds and stir. Sprinkle in the salt and mix again.
5. Spread the almonds evenly on the prepared baking dish and place in the oven.
6. Cook for 45 minutes, stirring well every 10 minutes.
7. Once cooked, transfer the nuts to paper towels to drain. When cool, store in an airtight container until ready to serve.

PER SERVING (ABOUT 27)

Calories: 305|Fat: 25g|Protein: 10g|Total carbs: 10g|Net carbs: 4g|Fiber: 6g|Fat: 74%|Protein: 13%|Carbs: 13%

Banana "Nice" Cream

Prep time: 5 minutes|Cooking time:10 minutes|Serves 8

- 4 frozen, diced bananas

1. In a food processor or blender, blend the bananas for 3 to 5 minutes until they reach a whipped, creamy consistency.
2. Depending on how frozen the bananas are, it may take a bit longer.
3. Serve immediately.

PER SERVING

Calories 112| Total Fat 0g| Saturated Fat 0g| Cholesterol 0mg| Carbohydrates 29g| Fiber 3g| Protein 1g

Mediterranean Cucumber Bites

Prep time: 10 minutes | Cook time: 15 minutes | Serves 8

- 8 ounces cream cheese, at room temperature
- 2 tablespoons chopped flat-leaf parsley
- ⅓ cup diced black olives
- 1 bell pepper, diced
- 2 cucumbers, halved lengthwise and seeded
- 2 tablespoons sliced scallions

1. In a small bowl, mix together the cream cheese, parsley, olives, and bell pepper.
2. Fill each cucumber cavity with the cream cheese mixture. Sprinkle with the scallions, slice into 1-inch pieces, and serve.

PER SERVING (½ CUCUMBER)

Calories: 253|Fat: 21g|Protein: 6g|Total carbs: 10g|Net carbs: 8g|Fiber: 2g|Sugar: 4g|Sodium: 271mg Macros: Fat: 75%|Protein: 9%|Carbs: 16%

Parmesan Zucchini Chips

Serves 2 / Prep time: 20 minutes | Cook time: 20 minutes | Serves 4

- Nonstick cooking spray
- 2 medium zucchini, cut into ¼-inch coins
- ½ teaspoon salt
- 1 cup grated Parmesan cheese
- 1 teaspoon garlic powder
- ½ cup low-sugar marinara sauce

1. Preheat the oven to 425°F. Spray a baking sheet with cooking spray.
2. Put the zucchini slices in a medium bowl and sprinkle with the salt. Set aside for 15 minutes.
3. In a separate bowl, combine the Parmesan cheese and garlic powder.
4. Blot the zucchini with a paper towel and place on the prepared baking sheet.
5. Sprinkle each zucchini coin with a generous amount of the cheese mixture.
6. Bake for 15 to 20 minutes, or until the cheese topping is bubbling.
7. Serve with the marinara sauce for dipping.

PER SERVING

Calories: 249|Fat: 13g|Protein: 21g|Total carbs: 12g|Net carbs: 9g|Fiber: 3g|Sugar: 5g|Sodium: 1201mg Macros: Fat: 47%|Protein: 34%|Carbs: 19%

Roasted Cauliflower Hummus

Prep time: 20 minutes | Cook time: 40 minutes | Serves 6

- Nonstick cooking spray
- 1 pound cauliflower florets
- 4 or 5 garlic cloves, peeled but left whole
- ⅓ cup olive oil
- 1 tablespoon freshly squeezed lemon juice
- ½ teaspoon salt
- 1 teaspoon ground cumin
- ½ teaspoon paprika
- ¼ cup water

1. Preheat the oven to 400°F. Line a baking sheet with aluminum foil. Spray with nonstick cooking spray.
2. Place the florets and garlic on the prepared baking sheet. Drizzle with half the olive oil and toss well.
3. Bake for 35 to 40 minutes, or until the vegetables are very tender but not too crispy. Remove from the oven.
4. In a food processor or high-powered blender, combine the florets, garlic, lemon juice, salt, cumin, and paprika. Blend until the mixture forms a smooth purée. While the mixture is blending, pour in the remaining olive oil. Thin out the mixture with water, as needed, until you reach the desired consistency.
5. Transfer the hummus to a bowl and serve.

PER SERVING

Calories: 136|Fat: 12g|Protein: 2g|Total carbs: 5g|Net carbs: 3g|Fiber: 2g|Sugar: 2g|Sodium: 218mg Macros: Fat: 79%|Protein: 6%|Carbs: 15%

No-Fail Deviled Eggs

Prep time: 20 minutes | Cook time: 15 minutes | Serves 8

- 8 hardboiled eggs
- 3 tablespoons veganaise
- 3 tablespoons relish
- 1 teaspoon Dijon mustard
- 1 teaspoon apple cider vinegar
- Paprika

1. Cut each egg in half vertically and scoop out the yolks. Place the yolks in a small bowl.
2. Add the veganaise, relish, mustard, and apple cider vinegar and mash well.
3. Use a spatula to scrape the yolk mixture into a sandwich-size plastic bag, and cut a small triangle off one bottom corner of the bag. Squeeze about 1 tablespoon of yolk mixture into the hollow of each egg-white half.
4. Sprinkle each egg half with paprika.
5. Arrange the eggs on a serving dish and serve immediately.

PER SERVING (2 EGGS)

Calories: 118|Fat: 9g|Protein: 6g|Total carbs: 3g|Net carbs: 3g|Fiber: 0g|Sugar: 2g|Sodium: 174mg Macros: Fat: 67%|Protein: 20%|Carbs: 13%

Flaxseed Chips And Guacamole

Prep time: 10 minutes | **Cook time:** 60 minutes | **Serves 6**

- 1 cup whole flaxseeds
- ½ cup vegetable broth
- 2 teaspoons garlic powder
- 2 teaspoons paprika
- 2 teaspoons onion powder
- 1 teaspoon onion salt
- 3 large avocados, halved
- ½ cup diced red onion
- 1 tablespoon freshly squeezed lime juice
- ½ teaspoon salt
- ¼ teaspoon ground cumin

1. Preheat the oven to 325°F. Line a baking sheet with parchment paper.
2. In a large mixing bowl, combine flaxseeds, broth, garlic powder, paprika, onion powder, and onion salt, and mix well.
3. Spread into a thin, even layer on the prepared baking sheet and bake for 55 to 60 minutes.
4. While the chips are baking, mash the avocado in a medium mixing bowl.
5. Mix in the red onion, lime juice, salt, and cumin. Cover the bowl and place it in the refrigerator until you are ready to eat.
6. Remove the flaxseed chips from the oven and allow them to cool|then break them apart into chip-size pieces. Serve with the guacamole.

PER SERVING

Calories: 328|Fat: 24g|Protein: 8g|Total carbs: 20g|Net carbs: 5g|Fiber: 15g|Sugar: 2g|Sodium: 441mg Macros: Fat: 66%|Protein: 10%|Carbs: 24%

Zucchini Fritters

Prep time: 20 minutes | **Cook time:** 15 minutes | **Serves 8**

- 2 cups grated zucchini
- ½ teaspoon salt
- 2 eggs, beaten
- ½ teaspoon baking powder
- ½ cup almond flour
- 2 tablespoons coconut flour
- ¼ cup Parmesan cheese
- ½ cup peanut oil
- ½ cup sour cream
- 2 tablespoons chopped fresh chives

1. Line a plate with paper towels.
2. In a medium bowl, sprinkle the zucchini with the salt. Set aside for 5 minutes. Transfer the zucchini to a colander and squeeze it dry with more paper towels.
3. Once the zucchini is as dry as possible, return it to the bowl. Add the eggs, baking powder, almond flour, coconut flour, and Parmesan cheese. Mix until well combined and a batter forms. Set aside.
4. Pour the oil into a small skillet over high heat.
5. Using ¼ cup of batter per fritter, pour batter into the hot skillet and spread into flat pancakes. Cook for 3 minutes, flip, and cook for an additional 3 minutes. Transfer to the paper towel–lined plate to drain.
6. Repeat to make more fritters until all the batter has been used.
7. Serve each fritter topped with 1 tablespoon of sour cream and sprinkled with chives.

PER SERVING (1 FRITTER)

Calories: 166|Fat: 14g|Protein: 5g|Total carbs: 5g|Net carbs: 3g|Fiber: 2g|Sugar: 1g|Sodium: 207mg Macros: Fat: 76%|Protein: 12%|Carbs: 12%

Cheesy Crackers

Prep time: 15 minutes | **Cook time:** 30 minutes | **Makes 55 to 60 crackers**

- 6 ounces Parmesan cheese
- 1½ cups almond flour
- ½ teaspoon salt
- ½ teaspoon garlic powder
- 1 egg
- 2 tablespoons butter, melted

1. Preheat the oven to 300°F. Line a baking sheet with parchment paper.
2. In a medium, microwave-safe bowl, heat the Parmesan cheese in the microwave in 30-second increments until melted, stirring between each cycle.
3. Add the flour, salt, garlic powder, and egg to the cheese mixture. Stir quickly until a dough forms. If the batter seems too sticky, use additional almond flour until it is no longer sticky.
4. Place the dough on a floured surface (or on parchment paper), and roll out to an ⅛-inch thickness. Cut the dough into 1-inch squares and use a spatula to carefully transfer the crackers to the prepared baking sheet.
5. Brush the melted butter across the top of each cracker.
6. Bake the crackers for 25 to 30 minutes, or until the tops are slightly browned.
7. Remove from the oven and allow to cool.

PER SERVING (10 CRACKERS)

Calories: 256|Fat: 20g|Protein: 14g|Total carbs: 5g|Net carbs: 3g|Fiber: 2g|Sugar: 0g|Sodium: 501mg Macros: Fat: 70%|Protein: 22%|Carbs: 8%

Caprese Stuffed Avocados

Prep time: 10 minutes | Cook time: 10 minutes | Serves 6-8

- ½ cup small mozzarella balls or bocconcini
- ⅓ cup halved cherry tomatoes
- 2 tablespoons pesto
- 2 garlic cloves, minced
- 1 teaspoon garlic salt
- 2 avocados, halved
- 2 tablespoons balsamic vinegar
- Freshly ground black pepper
- 2 tablespoons chopped fresh basil

1. In a medium bowl, mix together the mozzarella, tomatoes, pesto, garlic, and garlic salt.
2. Fill each avocado half with one-fourth of the cheese-and-tomato mixture.
3. Drizzle with the vinegar, season with pepper, and garnish with the basil.
1. Cheesy Cauliflower Breadsticks make a nice, crunchy side for this dish.

PER SERVING (1 AVOCADO HALF)

Calories: 244|Fat: 20g|Protein: 6g|Total carbs: 10g|Net carbs: 4g|Fiber: 6g|Sugar: 2g|Sodium: 145mg Macros: Fat: 74%|Protein: 10%|Carbs: 16%

Baked Olives

Prep time: 5 minutes | Cook time: 30 minutes | Serves 8

- Nonstick cooking spray
- 1 (6-ounce) can black olives, drained
- 1 (6-ounce) jar green olives, drained
- 14 ounces feta cheese, crumbled
- 2 tablespoons minced fresh rosemary
- 2 tablespoons minced fresh thyme
- 2 tablespoons olive oil

1. Preheat the oven to 350°F. Spray an 8-by-8-inch baking dish with cooking spray.
2. Pour the olives into the prepared dish. Stir in the feta cheese, rosemary, and thyme.
3. Drizzle the olive oil on top and mix well until the olives and cheese are well coated.
4. Bake for 22 to 25 minutes. Turn the oven to low broil and broil for an additional 2 to 4 minutes, or until the olives are browned.
5. Remove from the oven and serve warm.

PER SERVING

Calories: 284|Fat: 24g|Protein: 10g|Total carbs: 7g|Net carbs: 5g|Fiber: 2g|Sugar: 3g|Sodium: 1241mg Macros: Fat: 76%|Protein: 14%|Carbs: 10%

Savory Party Mix

Prep time: 5 minutes | Cook time: 20 minutes | Serves 12

- ½ cup pecans
- ½ cup cashews
- ½ cup pistachios
- ½ cup peanuts
- ½ cup almonds
- ½ cup pumpkin seeds
- 2 teaspoons onion powder
- 1 teaspoon garlic powder
- ½ teaspoon salt
- 2 tablespoons olive oil

1. Preheat the oven to 350°F. Line a baking sheet with parchment paper.
2. In a large mixing bowl, combine the pecans, cashews, pistachios, peanuts, almonds, pumpkin seeds, and sunflower seeds. Stir in the onion powder, garlic powder, and salt. Pour in the oil. Toss well to thoroughly coat the nuts and seeds with the oil.
3. Spread the mixture in a single layer on the prepared baking sheet and bake for 10 minutes. Stir well and place back in the oven to bake for 10 additional minutes.
4. Remove from the oven and allow to cool completely before serving.

PER SERVING (⅓ CUP)

Calories: 214|Fat: 18g|Protein: 6g|Total carbs: 7g|Net carbs: 5g|Fiber: 2g|Sugar: 1g|Sodium: 114mg Macros: Fat: 76%|Protein: 11%|Carbs: 13%

Three-Cheese Stuffed Mushrooms

Prep time: 10 minutes | Cook time: 15 minutes | Serves 6-8

- 12 button mushrooms, wiped clean and stems removed
- 1 tablespoon olive oil
- 4 ounces cream cheese
- ½ cup grated Parmesan cheese
- ½ cup grated Gruyère cheese
- 3 garlic cloves, minced
- 2 tablespoons chopped fresh parsley
- ¼ teaspoon garlic salt

1. Preheat the oven to 375°F. Line a baking sheet with parchment paper.
2. In a small bowl, toss the mushroom caps with the olive oil. Place the caps upside down on the prepared baking sheet.
3. In a separate small bowl, beat together the cream cheese, Parmesan cheese, Gruyère cheese, garlic, parsley, and garlic salt.
4. Fill each mushroom cap with the cheese mixture.
5. Bake for 15 minutes, and serve warm.

PER SERVING (3 MUSHROOMS)

Calories: 257|Fat: 21g|Protein: 12g|Total carbs: 5g|Net carbs: 4g|Fiber: 1g|Sugar: 1g|Sodium: 247mg Macros: Fat: 74%|Protein: 19%|Carbs: 7%

Creamy Spinach Dip

Prep time: 5 minutes | Cook time: 20 minutes | Serves 8

- Nonstick cooking spray
- 1 (10-ounce) package frozen spinach, thawed, drained, and squeezed dry
- 8 ounces cream cheese
- 8 ounces sour cream
- 2 tablespoons ranch seasoning
- ½ cup grated Parmesan cheese

1. Preheat the oven to 350°F. Spray an 8-by-8-inch baking dish with nonstick cooking spray. Set aside.
2. In a small bowl, mix together the spinach with the cream cheese and sour cream until well blended. Stir in the ranch seasoning.
3. Spread the mixture in the prepared baking dish and sprinkle with the Parmesan cheese.
4. Bake for 20 minutes, or until the cheese is melted.

PER SERVING

Calories: 259 | Fat: 23g | Protein: 8g | Total carbs: 5g | Net carbs: 4g | Fiber: 1g | Sugar: 0g | Sodium: 368mg Macros: Fat: 80% | Protein: 12% | Carbs: 8%

Herbed Mozzarella Sticks

Prep time: 10 minutes | Cook time: 20 minutes | Serves 8

- ½ cup peanut oil
- 1 cup very finely grated Parmesan cheese
- 1 tablespoon Italian seasoning
- ½ teaspoon garlic salt
- 8 sticks full-fat string cheese, halved horizontally
- 2 eggs, beaten

1. Pour the peanut oil into a small skillet over high heat. Line a plate with paper towels.
2. While the oil is heating, in a small bowl, mix together the grated Parmesan cheese, Italian seasoning, and garlic salt.
3. Dredge each mozzarella stick first in the beaten egg and then in the cheese-and-herb mixture, rolling the sticks so they are fully coated.
4. Carefully slip 3 or 4 sticks into the hot oil. Cook until all sides are golden brown, about 3 minutes.
5. Transfer to the paper towel–lined plate to drain for a few minutes.
6. Repeat with the remaining cheese sticks, and serve warm.

PER SERVING (2 STICKS)

Calories: 425 | Fat: 33g | Protein: 28g | Total carbs: 4g | Net carbs: 4g | Fiber: 0g | Sugar: 1g | Sodium: 623mg Macros: Fat: 70% | Protein: 26% | Carbs: 4%

Cheesy Cauliflower Breadsticks

Prep time: 25 minutes | Cook time: 35 minutes | Serves 8

- 1 head cauliflower, chopped into florets
- 4 egg whites
- ½ cup grated sharp cheddar cheese, divided
- ½ cup grated Parmesan cheese, divided
- 1 teaspoon dried oregano
- ¼ teaspoon salt

1. Preheat the oven to 450°F. Line a baking sheet with parchment paper.
2. Put the cauliflower florets in a food processor and pulse until the florets are as small as grains of rice.
3. Transfer the cauliflower to a microwave-safe bowl and cook in the microwave for 7 minutes. Remove and allow to cool for 5 minutes.
4. Pour the cooked cauliflower into a cheesecloth or clean kitchen towel and squeeze to remove as much moisture as possible. The drier the cauliflower, the better the result.
5. In a medium mixing bowl, combine the cauliflower, egg whites, ¼ cup of the cheddar cheese, ¼ cup of Parmesan cheese, oregano, and salt. Mix until a dough forms.
6. Place the dough on top of the parchment paper on the baking sheet. Use a rolling pin to roll it out into a rectangle or circle about ¼ inch thick.
7. Cook the cauliflower crust for 16 to 18 minutes or until light golden brown.
8. Remove the baking sheet from the oven and top the crust with the remaining ¼ cup of cheddar and ¼ cup of Parmesan cheese. Bake for an additional 5 minutes. Turn the oven to low broil and broil for 3 minutes, or until the cheese is bubbling.
9. Remove from the oven, cut into 12 breadsticks, and serve warm.

PER SERVING (2 BREADSTICKS)

Calories: 93 | Fat: 5g | Protein: 9g | Total carbs: 3g | Net carbs: 2g | Fiber: 1g | Sugar: 1g | Sodium: 277mg Macros: Fat: 48% | Protein: 39% | Carbs: 13%

Appendix 1 Measurement Conversion Chart

Volume Equivalents (Dry)	
US STANDARD	METRIC (APPROXIMATE)
1/8 teaspoon	0.5 mL
1/4 teaspoon	1 mL
1/2 teaspoon	2 mL
3/4 teaspoon	4 mL
1 teaspoon	5 mL
1 tablespoon	15 mL
1/4 cup	59 mL
1/2 cup	118 mL
3/4 cup	177 mL
1 cup	235 mL
2 cups	475 mL
3 cups	700 mL
4 cups	1 L

Volume Equivalents (Liquid)		
US STANDARD	US STANDARD (OUNCES)	METRIC (APPROXIMATE)
2 tablespoons	1 fl.oz.	30 mL
1/4 cup	2 fl.oz.	60 mL
1/2 cup	4 fl.oz.	120 mL
1 cup	8 fl.oz.	240 mL
1 1/2 cup	12 fl.oz.	355 mL
2 cups or 1 pint	16 fl.oz.	475 mL
4 cups or 1 quart	32 fl.oz.	1 L
1 gallon	128 fl.oz.	4 L

Weight Equivalents	
US STANDARD	METRIC (APPROXIMATE)
1 ounce	28 g
2 ounces	57 g
5 ounces	142 g
10 ounces	284 g
15 ounces	425 g
16 ounces (1 pound)	455 g
1.5 pounds	680 g
2 pounds	907 g

Temperatures Equivalents	
FAHRENHEIT(F)	CELSIUS(C) APPROXIMATE)
225 °F	107 °C
250 °F	120 ° °C
275 °F	135 °C
300 °F	150 °C
325 °F	160 °C
350 °F	180 °C
375 °F	190 °C
400 °F	205 °C
425 °F	220 °C
450 °F	235 °C
475 °F	245 °C
500 °F	260 °C

Appendix 2 The Dirty Dozen and Clean Fifteen

The Environmental Working Group (EWG) is a nonprofit, nonpartisan organization dedicated to protecting human health and the environment Its mission is to empower people to live healthier lives in a healthier environment. This organization publishes an annual list of the twelve kinds of produce, in sequence, that have the highest amount of pesticide residue-the Dirty Dozen-as well as a list of the fifteen kinds of produce that have the least amount of pesticide residue-the Clean Fifteen.

THE DIRTY DOZEN	
The 2016 Dirty Dozen includes the following produce. These are considered among the year's most important produce to buy organic:	
Strawberries	Spinach
Apples	Tomatoes
Nectarines	Bell peppers
Peaches	Cherry tomatoes
Celery	Cucumbers
Grapes	Kale/collard greens
Cherries	Hot peppers
The Dirty Dozen list contains two additional items kale/collard greens and hot peppers-because they tend to contain trace levels of highly hazardous pesticides.	

THE CLEAN FIFTEEN	
The least critical to buy organically are the Clean Fifteen list. The following are on the 2016 list:	
Avocados	Papayas
Corn	Kiw
Pineapples	Eggplant
Cabbage	Honeydew
Sweet peas	Grapefruit
Onions	Cantaloupe
Asparagus	Cauliflower
Mangos	
Some of the sweet corn sold in the United States are made from genetically engineered (GE) seedstock. Buy organic varieties of these crops to avoid GE produce.	

Appendix 3 Index

A

all-purpose flour 50, 53
allspice 15
almond 5, 14
ancho chile 10
ancho chile powder 5
apple 9
apple cider vinegar 9
arugula 51
avocado 11

B

bacon 52
balsamic vinegar 7, 12, 52
basil 5, 8, 11, 13
beet 52
bell pepper 50, 51, 53
black beans 50, 51
broccoli 51, 52, 53
buns 52
butter 50

C

canola oil 50, 51, 52
carrot 52, 53
cauliflower 5, 52
cayenne 5, 52
cayenne pepper 52
Cheddar cheese 52
chicken 6
chili powder 50, 51
chipanle pepper 50
chives 5, 6, 52
cinnamon 15
coconut 6
Colby Jack cheese 51
coriander 52
corn 50, 51
corn kernels 50
cumin 5, 10, 15, 50, 51, 52

D

diced panatoes 50
Dijon mustard 7, 12, 13, 51
dry onion powder 52

E

egg 14, 50, 53
enchilada sauce 51

F

fennel seed 53
flour 50, 53
fresh chives 5, 6, 52
fresh cilantro 52
fresh cilantro leaves 52
fresh dill 5
fresh parsley 6, 52
fresh parsley leaves 52

G

garlic 5, 9, 10, 11, 13, 14, 50, 51, 52, 53
garlic powder 8, 9, 52, 53

H

half-and-half 50
hemp seeds 8
honey 9, 51

I

instant rice 51

K

kale 14
kale leaves 14
ketchup 53
kosher salt 5, 10, 15

L

lemon 5, 6, 14, 51, 53
lemon juice 6, 8, 11, 13, 14, 51
lime 9, 12
lime juice 9, 12
lime zest 9, 12

M

maple syrup 7, 12, 53
Marinara Sauce 5
micro greens 52
milk 5, 50
mixed berries 12
Mozzarella 50, 53
Mozzarella cheese 50, 53
mushroom 51, 52
mustard 51, 53
mustard powder 53

N

nutritional yeast 5

O

olive oil 5, 12, 13, 14, 50, 51, 52, 53
onion 5, 50, 51
onion powder 8
oregano 5, 8, 10, 50

P

panatoes 50, 52
paprika 5, 15, 52
Parmesan cheese 51, 53
parsley 6, 52
pesto 52
pink Himalayan salt 5, 7, 8, 11
pizza dough 50, 53
pizza sauce 50
plain coconut yogurt 6
plain Greek yogurt 5
porcini powder 53
potato 53

R

Ranch dressing 52
raw honey 9, 12, 13
red pepper flakes 5, 8, 14, 15, 51, 53
ricotta cheese 53

S

saffron 52
Serrano pepper 53
sugar 10
summer squash 51

T

tahini 5, 8, 9, 11
thyme 50
toasted almonds 14
tomato 5, 50, 52, 53
turmeric 15

U

unsalted butter 50
unsweetened almond milk 5

V

vegetable broth 50
vegetable stock 51

W

white wine 8, 11
wine vinegar 8, 10, 11

Y

yogurt 5, 6

Z

zucchini 50, 51, 52, 53

CATHERINE S. TAYLOR